GOLDEN TRANSITION

Menopause Made Easy through
Maharishi Vedic Medicine

OTHER BOOKS BY DR. KUMUDA REDDY:

Forever Healthy—Introduction to Maharishi Ayur-Veda Health Care
by Kumuda Reddy, M.D. and Stan Kendz

For a Blissful Baby: Healthy and Happy Pregnancy with Maharishi Vedic Medicine
by Kumuda Reddy, M.D., Linda Egenes, M.A. and Margaret Mullins, MSN, CFNP.

All Love Flows to the Self: Eternal Stories from the Upanishads
by Kumuda Reddy, M.D., Thomas Egenes and Linda Egenes

Conquering Chronic Disease
by Kumuda Reddy, M.D. and Linda Egenes, M.A.

His Holiness Maharishi Mahesh Yogi: A Living Saint for the New Millenium
told by Helena and Roland Olson

The *Timeless Wisdom* Series of children's stories, by Kumuda Reddy, M.D. and John Pruitt:

The Indigo Jackal
The Lion and the Hare
The Monkey and the Crocodile
The Female Mouse
The Hares and the Elephants

At your bookstore or from the publisher:
Lantern Books/Samhita Productions
1 Union Square West Suite 201
New York, NY 10003
212-414-2275
www.lanternbooks.com
www.allhealthyfamily.com

GOLDEN TRANSITION

Menopause Made Easy through Maharishi Vedic Medicine

by
Kumuda Reddy, M.D.
and
Janardhan Reddy, M.D.
with
Sandra Willbanks, M.A.

Samhita Productions
Schenectady, New York

All illustrations courtesy of Kathryn Peckman, Jo Ann Gessner and Craig Ridgley

Published by Lantern Books
1 Union Square West, Suite 201, New York, New York 10003

ISBN 1-930051-56-5

We gratefully acknowledge permission to use material from the following published sources. The charts and text on pages 20, 22, 24, 137, and 161 are adapted from *Scientific Research on the Maharishi Transcendental Meditation and TM-Sidhi Programs: A Brief Summary of 500 Studies* (Fairfield, IA: Maharishi University of Management Press), ©1996 by Maharishi University of Management, and from *Scientific Research on the Maharishi Technology of the Unified Field: The Transcendental Meditation and TM-Sidhi Program* (Fairfield, IA: Maharishi International University Press), ©1988 by Maharishi International University. The charts and text on pages 21, 143, and 187 are adapted from *Summary of Research Findings* (Colorado Springs, CO: Maharishi Ayur-Veda Products International, Inc.), 1996.

Printed in the United States of America.

To our parents with love and gratitude
Kameswaramma and Harischandra Reddy
and Susheela and Satyanarayana Reddy.

Dedication

To Maharishi Mahesh Yogi, for giving us his vision of natural and holistic health in all areas of our lives.

Table of Contents

Acknowledgements

We would like to thank Professor Tony Nader, M.D., Ph.D., Dr. Keith and Samantha Wallace, Vaidya Hemant Gupta and Dr. Veronica Butler for their guidance and wisdom throughout the writing of this book. Our gratitude also goes to Mary Zillbeck and Martha Bright for their editing skills, Kathryn Peckman for the pictures, Craig Ridgley for the graphics and to all others who have supported us in the production of this book.

Foreword

In *Golden Transition* Dr. Reddy has beautifully brought to light in easy to understand terms a natural and complete understanding of how a woman's physiology works. She gives you the key for prevention of problems at menopause, explains what creates imbalances in the physiology, the different stages of imbalances and simple ways of preventing them.

This book shatters the myth that the problems associated with menopause are connected to a disorder in the physiology and must be corrected only by drugs, such as hormone replacement therapy. As put forth in this book, Maharishi Vedic Medicine knows that these disorders are caused by *pragya-apradh* (mistake of the intellect) and are caused by a basic ignorance of what holistic routines need to be undertaken during the monthly cycle and during the transition into menopause. The approaches of Maharishi Vedic Medicine practiced during and before menopause are so natural that they enliven the body's own inner intelligence. Prescribing isolated hormones for menopause may be good in one area but can cause trouble in another by undesirable and unintended side-effects. The holistic approach of Maharishi Vedic Medicine brings wholeness and balances while enlivening the body's inner intelligence, and gives bliss, happiness and everlasting energy.

As Dr. Reddy so eloquently points out, the transition into menopause is very natural and not a "curse." It can be a very smooth transition if it is viewed as an expression of the organizing power of Natural Law. Natural Law is the natural unfoldment of the laws of nature that create the structure and function of the entire creation including the human body and the whole universe. Acting spontaneously in accord with Natural Law means spontaneously acting in a way that supports well-being. Ill health results from the disturbance of the normal sequence in the expression of Natural Law. If the life is in tune with the Natural Law then problems will not occur because daily life is guided spontaneously by the laws of nature. The wholeness of Maharishi Vedic Medicine automatically enlivens all the laws of nature, from the finest level of creation to the grossest level of creation.

By promoting balance in every area of life, physical, mental, behavioral, emotional and spiritual, a woman becomes in tune with who she truly is and understands how beautifully her body functions. Through the approaches of Maharishi Vedic Medicine—connecting to one's self at the level of consciousness through the practice of the Transcendental Meditation technique, understanding the effects of both the near and far environments, understanding the benefits of purification and rejuvenation techniques, getting proper nourishment, rest and exercise—all add in making the later wisdom years of a woman's life truly golden.

A side benefit of the knowledge contained in *Golden Transition* is that it not only helps with the transition into menopause but it also helps the woman who is still having her monthly cycle understand how to make it smooth and worry-free. All of the transitions in a woman's life, from puberty to having periods to the cessation of periods into menopause can go very smoothly by applying the principles contained in this extraordinary book.

Through the wealth of knowledge contained in *Golden Transition*, Dr. Reddy has made a great contribution in bringing an understanding of how menopause is really a golden transition in a woman's life. I highly recommend that every woman read this book and apply the knowledge to their benefit.

Vaidya Hemant Gupta, M.D. (Ayur-Veda)
Associate Professor at the College of Maharishi Vedic Medicine, Fairfield, IA.
Associate Director, Ph.D. Program — Human Physiology with emphasis in Maharishi Vedic Medicine at Maharishi University of Management, Fairfield, IA.

Preface

This book is not just for women who have problems during menopause, but for all women. We're in the same boat, you and me, flowing along the river of life. We're all in this together, facing the same challenges.

Some of my colleagues tell me that menopause is like a disease and that every woman needs hormone replacement therapy. I am here to tell you that menopause is not a disease. It is a natural change in the stage of life, like the seasons changing from summer to fall. Every season displays its own glory and splendor—and also brings its own chores. The midlife change is like that, a time in life with its own work to be done.

In my experience, many women go through menopause rather uneventfully. For those who do have problems, there is a wide range of experience, from minor discomfort to real and prolonged suffering. Some women experience hot flashes, headaches, skin rashes or acne, irritability, and an increase in appetite. Others experience weight gain, fluid retention, lethargy, depression and sleep disorders. Still others experience anxiety, fatigue, trouble with memory or concentration, genitourinary problems or difficulties with digestion. For many women, there are the added concerns of heart disease, osteoporosis and other degenerative diseases, loneliness and fear.

Maharishi Vedic Medicine recognizes that each woman responds differently to premenopause and menopause, and that any symptoms of discomfort are manifestations of underlying imbalances in the mind and body that have accumulated over time. This book will explain these imbalances in greater detail and tell you how to recognize them and how to treat them.

When we are dealing with such a broad range of possible symptoms, it is important to realize that prescription hormones and drugs are not the answer. Only multiple modalities using holistic therapies can address the situation. Maharishi Vedic Medicine is a complete system of natural medicine that addresses all levels of mind, body, emotions, behavior and environment.

To give just one example, phytoestrogens and progesterone are available naturally in many grains, legumes and vegetables. Maharishi Vedic Medicine gives special food guidelines, herbal formulas and other natural therapies that balance the functioning of the whole physiology, so that there is no need for hormone replacement therapy. Every approach of this medicine works from the inside out, to enliven a woman's biological intelligence so that she functions more in accord with all the laws of nature.

A woman is sensitive, intelligent and intuitive by nature. Maharishi Vedic Medicine honors and respects these qualities. It does not violate a woman's body with harsh treatment, unwanted side effects or unnatural ingredients. It works with nature to accomplish good health from within, in a balanced and nourishing way.

This system of medicine also recognizes that menopause is a beautiful period in a woman's life. Every woman is really a goddess in disguise, radiating beauty, wisdom and courage. The maturity and experience of midlife are strengths that can be developed even further. She can continue to grow in wisdom and become a blessing to herself, her family, her community and her world.

A lot can be accomplished quickly during times of change. For this reason, menopause is a precious opportunity. We can use this time to restructure our physiologies and change the direction of our lives. Menopause is not a disease, and it's not something to dwell upon. With Maharishi Vedic Medicine we can begin anywhere at any time, regain our health, and move on to fulfill our desires.

I invite you to enjoy this timely medicine and live in freedom—free from ill health, free from fear, free to enjoy growing peace, happiness, health and longevity.

Kumuda Reddy, M.D.
Bethesda, Maryland
May, 2003

Introduction to Maharishi Vedic Medicine

The goal of any system of health care, to create healthy individuals and a disease-free society, can be achieved only through complete knowledge of Natural Law—the principles forming the total organizing power of Nature responsible for the whole manifest universe. Until now medical practice has been limited in its effectiveness and dangerous in its side effects because it only makes use of isolated Laws of Nature.

Maharishi Vedic Medicine℠, based on total knowledge of Natural Law (Veda), has as its fundamental principle that in order to prevent sickness and disease, the inner intelligence of every aspect of the physiology must be maintained in its full alertness, its full vitality.

This inner intelligence consists of the fundamental structures of Natural Law—the 40 aspects of Veda and the Vedic Literature—which govern human physiology and the whole universe. The profound and practical application of this knowledge to health helps to bring all aspects of individual life into harmony with Natural Law—the basis for maintaining health and creating a disease-free society.

Over 600 scientific research studies, conducted at 200 universities and research institutes in 30 countries, document the benefits of certain programs of Maharishi Vedic Medicine for improved physiological, psychological, social and environmental health.

The Field of Intelligence at the Basis of Health

Maharishi Vedic Medicine approaches the problems of prevention and cure from the source of health, the most fundamental field of intelligence in Nature—known in modern science as the unified field—which governs every level of existence, from subatomic particles, to the human body, to the galactic universe. It is the lack of integration between the individual's physiology and this underlying field of intelligence that causes disorder and disease.

All the specific programs, procedures and technologies used in Maharishi Vedic Medicine help restore this integration to create a balanced state of health—perfect synchrony between the functioning of every individual cell and the holistic functioning of the whole body, and between the holistic intelligence of the body and cosmic intelligence, which is managing the orderly evolution of the universe without a problem.

Discovery of the Total Intelligence of Natural Law in Human Physiology

Maharishi Vedic Medicine has been revived at this time by the profound insights into the total knowledge of Natural Law brought to light by Maharishi Mahesh Yogi over the past 40 years. Based on Maharishi's work in the field of consciousness, Professor Tony Nader, M.D., Ph.D. discovered that the different aspects of human physiology form an exact replica of the patterns of intelligence expressed in the impulses of sound in Veda and Vedic Literature.

Veda and the Vedic Literature, expressing the total potential of Natural Law, are the "blueprints" for understanding human physiology—from the profound level of DNA as the first expression of intelligence in the body, to the cells and tissues, to the organs and autonomic systems structuring the whole physiology—and the relationship of individual life to society, to the environment and even to the extended environments of the cosmos.

Hazards of Modern Medicine

Everywhere in the world today medical experts and the general public are recognizing the limitations and hazards of the prevailing system of health care. This means that the knowledge and approaches being taught in conventional medical education are incomplete and even dangerous. As reported in the *Journal of the American Medical Association*, 100 million Americans, or nearly 40 percent of the population, suffer from chronic diseases. This is clear evidence of this incomplete knowledge.

The greatest threats to health—cardiovascular disease, cancer, other chronic diseases, accidents and violence—are caused or influenced by mental, behavioral or environmental factors not effectively understood or addressed by modern medicine.

The hazards of modern medicine have been documented in over 7,000 scientific articles published in the medical literature reporting the harmful and often fatal effects of drugs and other modern medical interventions. An article in the April 1998 issue of the *Journal of the American Medical Association* stated that modern medical procedures are themselves one of the major causes of death in the United States.

From the perspective of Maharishi Vedic Medicine, any failures of modern medicine result from one fundamental weakness: an isolated approach to knowledge and practice which fails to attend to the balance and integration of the physiology as a whole.

In contrast, Maharishi Vedic Medicine enlivens the inner intelligence of the physiology and restores the integration of this inner intelligence with the body to bring increasing balance to every aspect of health. This approach of Natural Law–based medicine is so comprehensive that treatment of any specific part promotes the health of the whole.

Maharishi Vedic Medicine Brings Completeness to Health Care

The effectiveness of Maharishi Vedic Medicine lies in the ability of its programs to enliven the total intelligence of Natural Law within the physiology, and thereby integrate the functioning of all aspects of body and mind. As a result, thought, action and behavior become more integrated and balanced, and spontaneously more in harmony with Natural Law, which is the basis of good health.

To fully enliven the connection between the body and its inner intelligence, Maharishi Vedic Medicine utilizes the knowledge contained in the 40 areas of Veda and the Vedic Literature. This holistic knowledge of Natural Law is uniquely applied for prevention and treatment of disease. It includes the following elements, which are not available in any other medical system:

Veda and Vedic Literature in Human Physiology

Maharishi Vedic Medicine brings to light the fundamental structures of Natural Law contained in Veda and the Vedic Literature and the precise relationship between the structure and functions of human physiology. Maharishi Vedic Medicine understands how these 40 areas of Natural Law administer all aspects of the physiology at its most basic level and are included in the complete consideration of health.

Pulse Diagnosis

This is a method to detect balance and imbalance in the body by feeling the pulse and restoring balance before disease arises. By using this particular method of pulse reading, a physician trained in Maharishi Vedic Medicine can detect current and future imbalances and determine the healthiest **diet**, **daily** and **seasonal routines**, and **herbal preparations** for your specific mind-body system. Pulse diagnosis is an extremely effective diagnostic tool because it can help the physician detect imbalances before they develop into full-blown symptoms.

Vedic Sounds

These vibrations of the field of pure intelligence are used to restore balance to the physiology.

Vedic Architecture (Maharishi Sthapatya Veda℠ design)

These are ancient principles for designing and constructing

buildings according to Natural Law for the health, happiness and good fortune of the inhabitants. According to this science, health is profoundly influenced by the orientation and shape of buildings and land.

Vedic system of predicting the future (Maharishi Jyotish℠ program)

By understanding the relationship between human physiology and its cosmic counterparts (the far-distant environment) one can avert potential problems and promote positive trends in health and all aspects of life. The relationship of human physiology and the cosmos is evident in the diurnal, monthly and seasonal cycles that affect chemical, hormonal and other processes in the physiology. Professor Tony Nader's discovery brings to light the profound and precise connections between the structures of human physiology and the structures of the cosmos.

Maharishi Transcendental Meditation℠ and TM-Sidhi® programs

These programs, including Yogic Flying, give direct experience of the total field of intelligence and promote deep rest, release stress and develop a high level of mind-body coordination. Hundreds of research studies show the benefits of this technology for mind, body, behavior and environment.

Improved Collective Health

The practice of these technologies of consciousness in large groups purifies collective consciousness and promotes positive trends in the whole society. Many large-scale research studies demonstrate that group practice of the TM-Sidhi program, including Yogic Flying, reduces negative social trends such as crime, accidents and disease, creating a powerful influence of coherence and harmony known as the Maharishi Effect.

Forty Approaches are Forty Aspects of Natural Law, as Contained in the Veda and Vedic Literature

In describing the Maharishi Vedic Approach to Health℠, sometimes various branches of the Vedic Literature are mentioned. For example, the Maharishi Vedic Astrology program comes from the knowledge of the aspect of the Vedic Literature called Jyotish, and Maharishi Sthapatya Veda design comes from the aspect called Sthapatya Veda.

There are forty aspects of the Vedic Literature; together, they express the knowledge of all the fundamental structures of Natural Law in the universe. Maharishi Vedic Medicine offers knowledge drawn from all forty aspects of the Vedic Literature-because they apply to health and well-being in every area of human life.

Based on Maharishi's insights into the Veda and Vedic Literature, Professor Tony Nader, M.D., Ph.D., an MIT-trained neuroscientist, has recently discovered that the different aspects of the human physiology form an exact replica of the patterns of intelligence that are expressed in the forty aspects of the Veda and Vedic Literature. This discovery reveals that the inner intelligence of the body, which governs all functions in the human physiology, is in actuality the same Laws of Nature that govern the entire universe. There is a saying from the Vedic Literature that expresses this idea in a simple way. It says, "As is the individual, so is the universe. As is the microcosm, so is the macrocosm" (*Charaka Samhita*, Sharirasthana 4:13).

This recognition- that the total range of Natural Law that constitutes the Veda is the same Natural Law expressed in our human consciousness, mind and body- helps modern science to bridge the gap between the individual, the environment and the universe. And even more importantly, this knowledge demonstrates that it is possible to treat the body completely from the level of the total intelligence of Natural Law. In other words, if we enliven the total potential of Natural Law at the basis of the physiology, the whole body can be transformed. If we awaken Nature's intelligence in the body, we can create ideal health.

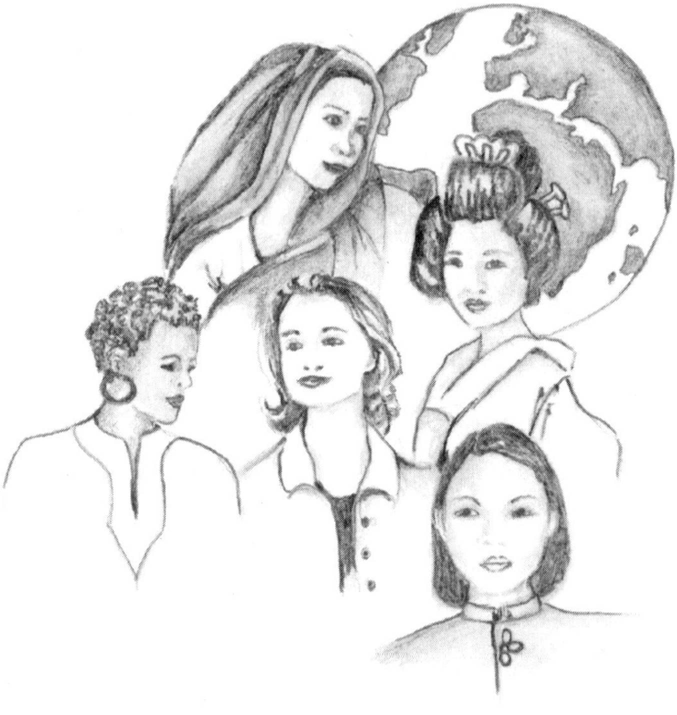

Chapter One

A Complete and Natural Approach to Menopause

Janet[1] was fifty when she started having delayed periods, hot flashes, high blood pressure and fatigue. She was experiencing a lot of stress and extreme anxiety during her work as a computer programmer, and with the addition of hot flashes, mostly during the night, she couldn't sleep. She was also having digestive problems.

Janet was told by her gynecologist that she was approaching menopause and that she would need hormone replacement therapy (HRT). But Janet was allergic to many conventional medicines and was afraid to go on HRT. She tried taking some herbal remedies prescribed by a naturopath, but was having only marginal relief. That's when she tried Maharishi Vedic Medicine.

Like most of the women who come to see me* at the onset of menopause, Janet had numerous complaints. That is why the natural approach of Maharishi Vedic Medicine works so well, because, unlike allopathic medicine, which tends to use a one-drug-per-symptom approach, Maharishi Vedic Medicine presents a holistic system of natural health care. By focusing on the underlying physiological imbalances that give rise to symptoms of disease, Maharishi Vedic Medicine can address a whole gamut of diverse symptoms with recommendations tailored to each individual's specific concerns.

---

* The "I" in this book represents Dr. Kumuda Reddy's voice.

As part of the recommendations of Maharishi Vedic Medicine, Janet started a diet tailored to her individual needs. She also began taking specific herbal supplements for menopausal women and began practicing Maharishi Yoga℠ asanas. Most importantly, she started a program for relaxation and stress management known as the Transcendental Meditation® technique.

Within a month, Janet felt much better. Once she experienced less anxiety and more energy, Janet was able to deal with her work in a more productive and happier way. Then she was able to focus more on her physical and mental health and took a series of purification and rejuvenation treatments at a Maharishi Ayur-Veda Health Center. That's when Janet realized that she felt better than she had in years. Her weariness, despondency and exhaustion had given way to a youthful vivaciousness and her voice was full of energy.

She told me, "When I was feeling ill I couldn't find any fun in life or in my job. After following your recommendations I realized that I had been dragging this body around for years without experiencing the real spark of health."

Alice, a credit analyst for a bank, came to me with a different set of complaints. At age 46 she was perimenopausal with ups and downs in her energy level. With frequent bladder infections, she had been on repeated antibiotics to treat the condition, which in turn gave her repeated candida infections. In association with the bladder infection she also had diarrhea and experienced bloating after eating. In addition, she gained weight in the last three years which made her feel embarrassed and uncomfortable.

In the preceding two weeks before coming to see me, Alice frequently experienced heartburn and an uncomfortable hot feeling in her body. "I used to wear regular, medium-weight clothes," she said. "But now I sweat even wearing the lightest cotton."

All of these problems were fairly easy to resolve with the approaches of Maharishi Vedic Medicine, because the focus is on the entire patient and treating her from the source of her problems and not the symptoms themselves. Since she already practiced the Transcendental Meditation technique, I simply made changes in her diet and exercise program accompanied with Maharishi Ayur-Veda® herbal recommendations. I put her on a weight loss program that was right for her body's needs and addressed her various concerns about menopause.

In just a few weeks of incorporating this holistic approach, supported by her understanding of what was going on in her physiology, most of Alice's symptoms were better or had disappeared and she had lost some weight. I advised her to continue using the methods of Maharishi Vedic Medicine health care for one year so that all of these problems could be eliminated. Six months after she saw me she took Maharishi Ayur-Veda purification and rejuvenation treatments, which she later told me gave her great relief. In the last two years she hasn't had any recurring episodes of bladder infections or diarrhea.

Preparing for Menopause

If you are concerned about the possible negative affects of menopause, you are not alone. According to the North American Menopause Society, 4,000 women in the United States are reaching menopause every day. You may have only a vague idea of what to expect, and that idea may be based on what the media wants you to know.

Drug advertisers have a tendency to scare you into thinking that at the moment of menopause your bones will fracture at the slightest touch, you'll lose your feminine attractiveness overnight, and hot flashes will ruin your day. But you need to understand that what is going on in your physiology far outweighs the instant fix offered by drugs or surgery.

It is a myth that you can't prepare for menopause. You can and should.

With 38 million female baby boomers beginning the second

half of their lives, information is needed to make this a smooth, natural and evolutionary transition.

Menopause, Perimenopause and Post-Menopause

Menopause is the end of menstruation, the cyclical ovarian process that begins in puberty. Technically, menopause is the *point* at which your monthly menses stop and don't start again—which, as Germaine Greer points out in *The Change, Women, Aging and the Menopause,* is a non-event, because nothing actually happens.[2] Nothing happens but you might not realize it, if you have been experiencing stop-and-go periods. The word "menopause" has been used to cover both perimenopause, which happens before and just after the point of menopause, and post-menopause which starts a year after that point. Generally, menopause occurs as early as age 35, most often at age 50 or 51 and as late as age 55. Menopause is only one event in the *climacteric,* which is the biological change in all body tissue and systems that occurs in both sexes somewhere between the ages of 40 and 60.

Menopause affects each woman differently. This rite of passage is made easily by approximately 15 percent of women. They move without incident from the perimenopausal years to the post-menopausal years. Another 15 percent have a difficult time and need to take extra measures to feel healthy again. In the middle of these two groups is the largest group—70 percent—of women who don't have a sickness, but don't feel really great either.

The word "menopause" is two Greek words combined meaning "month" and "end," or the end of the monthly cycle. It comes from a monograph about the change of life written in 1812 by C. P. L. Gardanne, a French gynecologist. In his writings, Gardanne combined the two Greek words to form the word *menepausie.*[3]

Menopause occurs when the ovaries stop producing large amounts of estrogen and progesterone, two hormones intimately involved in the menstrual cycle. Many in today's medical community tend to view this process as an ailment—an unhealthy state of deficiency. This is because certain diseases have been shown to be related to the lack of hormones in a woman's body. For example, osteoporosis, the loss of density in the bones, can occur more quickly. Also, blood levels of cholesterol and triglycerides often start increasing, so that women become more prone to heart disease.

Perimenopause is a term used to define the upcoming change—heavy or lighter than usual menstrual periods, mood swings, headaches, fatigue, weight gain and other signs that estrogen and progesterone levels are in flux. The perimenopause years are the years just before and just after your last menstrual period. "Peri" means "surrounding"—that is why it is used instead of "pre," which means "before." The medical profession commonly refers to the irregular or heavy menstrual bleeding that may occur at this age as *perimenopausal bleeding.*

Post-menopause starts "officially" a year after your menstrual flow has stopped. Most of the time when people refer to menopause they are really talking about post-menopause.

Surgical Menopause

Premenopausal women who have both their ovaries removed surgically experience an abrupt menopause. They may be hit harder by menopausal symptoms than are those who experience it naturally, because their bodies have difficulty adjusting to such an abrupt change. Their hot flashes may be more severe, more frequent, and last longer. They may have a greater risk of heart disease and osteoporosis, and may be more prone to depression.

When only one ovary is removed, menopause usually occurs naturally. When the uterus is removed (hysterectomy) and the ovaries remain, menstrual periods stop but other menopausal symptoms (if any) usually occur at the same age that they would naturally. However, some women who have a hysterectomy may experience menopausal symptoms at a younger age.

Choosing a Natural Approach to Menopause

Recent studies have shown that hormone replacement therapy used for estrogen loss does not reduce the risk of developing heart disease.[4] In addition research has shown that side effects of HRT include uterine cancer, migraines, fibroid tumors and elevated blood pressure.

Nancy Lonsdorf, M.D. and Veronica Butler, M.D., co-authors of *A Woman's Best Medicine: Health, Happiness, and Long Life Through Ayur-Veda,*[5] stress that, "Nature didn't intend that women have the same amount of hormones throughout their life in order to stay healthy." From the point of view of the Maharishi Vedic Medicine program, the loss of estrogen merely sheds light on underlying imbalances that become noticeable when the added protection of estrogen is gone. If your physiology is balanced, you can have a comfortable menopause.

Early literature about menopause overemphasized the fact that menopause marks the end of a woman's reproductive years. Unfortunately, this implies that the years following menopause are "nonproductive." Advice is often given to take more hormones, get a hysterectomy, use drugs for the rest of your life. We have a health-care system that is really a disease-care system, spending one-tenth of its resources on preventing disease and nine-tenths on managing it.

Menopause is not a disease, it is simply a change. Change can create or point out an imbalance in the physiology that needs correcting. These corrections can be made through alternative approaches that directly address any discomfort during menopause.

Change in a positive direction is evolution. At menopause and post-menopause your body is evolving into an evolutionary phase that is designed by nature to be full of creativity, wisdom, health and happiness. Menopause is nature's way of telling you that, after a lifetime of focusing on others, it's time to focus on yourself; from there you can focus on your world family. It is inevitable that the changes that occur at menopause can bring on other changes in the body as well. Menopause signals the ideal time for you to inventory your health and make plans to follow the advice given for changes in a not-quite-so-healthy lifestyle.

Because Maharishi Vedic Medicine does not look at menopause as a disease, it does not suggest that everyone who has the same symptoms receive the same treatment. With the Maharishi Vedic Medicine program described in this book, you will have a complete, natural and practical system to make this time of change in your life comfortable and healthy. Please note, this book is not a substitute for professional medical treatment, but offers insight into different types of choices you can make. With the wisdom gained you just might ask yourself, "Why wasn't I doing this before?"

A Brief Overview of Maharishi Vedic Medicine

Maharishi Vedic Medicine is a holistic approach to health that covers all ages and aspects of one's life, environment and society. It is a practical guide that covers the physical, mental, emotional and spiritual aspects—the original approach to the mind-body connection. While Western medicine focuses solely on identifying and eliminating the isolated symptoms, Maharishi Vedic Medicine seeks to identify the underlying source that is the cause of so many symptoms. By eliminating the deep underlying imbalances, rather than the superficial symptoms, Maharishi Vedic Medicine provides much more effective methods to provide long-lasting and real relief from these problems. In other words, it takes into account the whole self and focuses first on developing the consciousness of the individual.

Veda is a Sanskrit word meaning knowledge. Maharishi Vedic Medicine is based on knowledge of the Veda. Veda itself cannot be bound within a book because it is not just the knowledge of facts, things or ideas. Rather, it is knowledge through direct experience of the abstract and all-inclusive field of consciousness itself.

You know when you've have the experience of simply knowing something to be true, even though you've never read anything about it or heard of the concept before? It just resonates somehow at a deep level. That kind of "knowing"—at the most deep and most profound level—is "Veda." Veda is pure knowledge, which was originally understood or "cognized" by the great seers of the ancient Vedic civilization in India. The classical Indian texts known collectively as the Vedic Literature are the written expression of this intelligence.

The *Charaka Samhita,* the *Sushruta Samhita,* and the *Ashtangas* are some of the oldest texts on *Ayur-Veda.* Ayur-Veda is formally recognized by the World Health Organization and is the traditional medical system of India.

The principles of Ayur-Veda are held to be immortal, having been understood through direct intuition by ancient sages or seers on the level of their own awareness. The ancient Vedic texts say that enlightened sages (*rishis*) became concerned about the ill health in the world and sought to uncover the deepest truths of human physiology so that suffering could be prevented. They meditated together in a large group while one of them, Bharadwaja, attempted to find the answer. In this coherent atmosphere, Bharadwaja cognized the essence of Ayur-Veda. It is considered the first organized approach to health and was put into written form by the physicians Charaka and Sushruta. Ayur-Veda is like a branch of the tree of Maharishi Vedic Medicine.

The other branches of Maharishi Vedic Medicine will be discussed later in this book. By having knowledge of all the aspects of Maharishi Vedic Medicine, you will be able to understand the whys and hows of living the next part of your life in an intelligent and wise manner.

Why Is This Health System Called Maharishi Vedic Medicine?

Over time and during the centuries of foreign rule in India, Ayurvedic institutions declined and much of Ayurvedic knowledge became misunderstood or lost. In recent decades, however, Ayurveda has undergone a remarkable resurgence. Most significantly, the collaboration of Maharishi Mahesh Yogi, founder of the Transcendental Meditation program, with leading Ayurvedic physicians throughout India known as *Vaidyas,* has resulted in the restoration of Ayurvedic approaches in accordance with the Vedic texts. The modern reformulation of this traditional health care system is known as the *Maharishi Ayur-Veda* health program in order to distinguish it from the fragmented version of Ayurveda which is still practiced in India and other countries today.

The "tree" of Maharishi Vedic Medicine is made up not only of the ancient Ayurvedic texts, but it includes all the aspects contained in the Veda and Vedic Literature as well. It is a complete health care system, effective in the areas of prevention of disease, preservation of health and the promotion of longevity. The primary goal of Maharishi Vedic Medicine is to increase the life span and improve the quality of life. The treatment and prevention of imbalances are important in achieving this goal.

The most accurate way to determine your state of balance is through a doctor trained in Maharishi Vedic Medicine (or Maharishi Ayur-Veda). Imbalances can be detected even before they manifest into symptoms. The doctor can then give you a list of recommendations, including meditation, proper diet, herbs, spices, exercise, yoga, daily and seasonal routines and rejuvenation therapies that correct the imbalances, put you back on the road to good health and let you feel comfortable in your body again. The advantage of this book is that it will give you good advice on health practices every woman can incorporate into her life right now.

In non-Western cultures, menopause does not carry the stigma that is associated with it in the West. Other cultures don't have the same problems. In a survey of menopausal symptoms in Japan it was found that the Japanese don't have a word for a hot flash.[6] The most common symptom menopausal Japanese woman had was stiff shoulders. Only 9.5 percent of women in Japan have what we in the west call hot flashes,[7] while between 50 to 80 percent of Western women have them.[8]

Mayan women have no symptoms of menopause, yet they have the same hormonal changes as women of other cultures.[9] They too have no word for a hot flash. Chinese women report few problems. A study by anthropologist Martha Frent looked at the Rajput women of Northern India. They had no symptoms of depression related to menopause because they view this time of their lives as freedom from menstruation, pregnancy and childbirth.[10]

The ancient texts of Ayur-Veda do not have a word for menopause. The texts do mention when the menses start and stop, but when the menses stop, then *Vata Kala*, or the time of wisdom, starts. This was never considered a problem but rather something to look forward to.

Problems at menopause experienced by women who live in industrialized nations are *abnormal* compared with women from other parts of the world who live a healthier lifestyle. When women come to me at menopause, they have a list of things that are going wrong in their physiology: headaches, body aches, insomnia, hot flashes, weight gain, depression and so forth. Unfortunately, one problem may be cleared up by one drug, but the other problems still exist. Sometimes the drug creates a problem of its own. Western treatments, more often than the general public is told, produce side effects. Some women who are simply looking for a way to feel well during their transition into menopause wind up in a hospital due to an illness "attributed to drugs."[11]

This sets up a cycle of going from one doctor to another to find a "cure." The doctors are not fully aware of each other's prescriptions, or what the patient has been doing. They especially don't know who the patient really is with respect to this holistic viewpoint and how she is going to react to specific suggestions.

Menopause is associated with *aging*, which in many cultures has negative associations. Aging relates to all sorts of things happening to your physiology.

What Causes Aging?

Modern science has not been able to determine exactly what causes aging. There are currently two major theories:

1. Aging is built into your genes. Your body is programmed to live only a biologically predetermined amount of time.
2. Symptoms of aging accumulate because your body doesn't repair and rebuild itself properly. Such errors cause wear and tear that leads to an eventual breakdown of life-support systems.

The Body Is a Self-Repairing Mechanism

The second theory is consistent with the knowledge of Maharishi Vedic Medicine, which can help you slow down the aging process by reducing wear and tear on the body. The purpose of Maharishi Vedic Medicine is, fundamentally, for a long and healthy life.

The innate intelligence for regenerating cells is encoded in your DNA, which gets passed from one generation of cells to the next. Your DNA contains the ability to repair itself if it gets damaged. Statistics now suggest that women in menopause have as long to live as they have already lived. Since the body is a self-repairing mechanism, if given the chance and the proper life-supporting ingredients, the body can maintain tiptop functioning for a very long time. With Maharishi Vedic Medicine, you have a choice as to how you are going to live the rest of your life.

Premature Aging and Free Radicals

The wear and tear of aging is related to free radical damage in the body. Free radicals are highly reactive oxygen molecules that cause oxidation—the process that makes metal rust, food grow moldy, and autumn leaves decay.

In your body, free radicals help to fight bacteria and remove toxins. Your body naturally produces substances such as superoxide dismutase (SOD) to keep free radicals in balance. But many factors of modern living generate an excessive amount of free radicals that can wreak havoc on your body—attacking healthy cells and tissues and even damaging your DNA. Due to stress and other factors, there are too many free radicals to control.

One of the obvious ways to prevent free radicals from running rampant in your body is to reduce the factors that cause them.

Factors that cause free radicals are:

- All types of mental and emotional stress
- Physical stress and extreme exertion—especially when you are not in shape
- Processed foods
- Foods grown with pesticides and herbicides
- Fatty foods such as meat, cheese, pastries
- Polyunsaturated and hydrogenated oils
- Alcoholic drinks
- Coffee
- Tobacco smoke
- Air and water pollution
- Ultraviolet rays from the sun or tanning lamps

Here is an interesting concept to grasp: aging is not fatal. You may have heard of someone dying of "natural causes"; but, the fact is that medical science has never documented that aging itself causes death. Rather, death is caused by a failure or defect in one of the central life-support systems. Your body's billions of cells are constantly replacing themselves—experiments at the Salk Institute for Biological Studies show evidence that even nerve cells in the brain rejuvenate, something not thought possible after a stroke, illness or injury (Nov. '98 *Journal of Natural Medicine*). There is no real reason for aging.

Although you never consciously realize it, your body is quietly producing a new stomach lining every five days, a new skin every five weeks, and new bones every three months. In Maharishi Vedic Medicine herbal formulations called *rasayanas* play a significant role in helping the body rejuvenate, increasing general immune system strength and promoting well-being. The importance of rasayanas is discussed in a later chapter.

If you choose it to be, menopause need not be the beginning of the end of your life but just the beginning of a healthier life. When you apply the principles of Maharishi Vedic Medicine to your life, you will not only have a smooth post-menopause, but you will also slow down the aging process. What a bonus! Who could have imagined such a profound side benefit to a treatment for menopause.

The First Step

So many of the women who come to see me have complaints of stress. Becky, 55, was complaining of anxiety with many panic attacks, especially when driving on highways. She had been put on medication for anxiety, but by the time I saw her she had become addicted to it and had been through a drug rehabilitation program to get off the drug. She was scared of taking any more unnatural medicine for her anxiety and panic attacks. She had other problems related to her fears, but the foremost recommendation to her was to learn to meditate.

Although the knowledge of how to live a healthy life is described in Vedic texts, the Maharishi Vedic Medicine approach states that all imbalance, all disease and disorder, is the loss of a natural, innate wisdom or consciousness that we have forgotten how to access. Mind and body are connected; and consciousness is part of both.

You have organizing principles of health within you; but they have been confused or overridden by the constant barrage of things to do, reasons to stay up late, eating on the run, all kinds of unnatural things that you are enticed to do. There is so much going on in the outside world that maybe you have forgotten how to access the inside world. The benefits of reawakening the naturally healthy state of being that resides inside you is enormous.

Remember in the list of factors that cause free radicals the first thing listed was all types of mental and emotional stress? This is something that cannot be completely avoided in our modern life. Even if we chose to live in an isolated woods somewhere, we would still have to deal with some type of stress. Just surviving can cause stress. You can't just think it away no matter how hard you try. Just *trying* to causes stress! What to do?

In order to *not* accumulate stress in the physiology, you have to dissolve it. The technique for eliminating stress is called the Transcendental Meditation (TM®) technique. This technique combined with the other health choices that you make will help tremendously with coping, living and loving the rest of your life.

The Transcendental Meditation technique is the most widely researched meditation technique in the world. There is no doubt that it works. It is an easily learned technique that gives deep rest to the mind and body, giving you a way to transcend the reasoning brain and enliven the physiology directly. This allows stress to dissolve. It also helps to coordinate mind-body function, which adds good-quality years to your life. This can happen even if your family history is not healthy. Your health is not dictated by your mother's health. You can change anything. You always have a choice.

References

1. All names in the case files are changed to protect privacy.

2. Greer, G. 1992. *The Change: Women, Aging and the Menopause.* New York: Alfred A. Knopf.
3. Jacobowitz, R.S. 1993. *150 Most Asked Questions About Menopause.* New York: William Morrow & Co., p. 41.
4. Gorman, C & Park, A. The Truth About Hormones. *Time* magazine. July 22, 2002.
5. Lonsdorf, Nancy, M.D., Butler, Veronica, M.D., and Brown, Melanie, Ph.D. 1993. *A Woman's Best Medicine: Health, Happiness and Long Life through Ayur-Veda.* New York: Tarcher/Putnam.
6. Lock, M., Kaufert, P. & Gilbert, P. 1988. Cultural construction of the menopausal syndrome: The Japanese case. *Maturitas,* 10, 317–332.
7. Lock, M.1994. Menopause in çultural context. *Experimental Gerontology,* 29(3/4), 307–317.
8. Kronenberg, F. & Downey, J.A. 1987 Thermoregulatory physiology of menopausal hot flashes: A review. *Canadian Journal of Physiological Pharmacology,* 65, 1312–24.
9. Martin, M.C., Block, J.E. Sanchez S.D, Arnaud, C.D. & Beyene, Y. 1993 Menopause without symptoms: The endocrinology of menopause among rural Mayan Indians. *American Journal of Obstetrics and Gynecology,* 168(6), 1839–1845.
10. Flint, M. & Samil R.S. 1986. Cultural and subcultural meanings of the menopause: A biocultural analysis. *Culture, Medicine and Psychiatry,* 10, 47–71.
11. Isselbacher, K.L., Braunwald, E., Wilson, J.D., Martin J.B., Fauci, A.S., Kasper D.L. (eds) 1994. *Harrison's Principles of Internal Medicine,* 13th ed. New York: McGraw-Hill, p. 405.

Chapter Two

The *Transcendental Meditation* Technique

One of the most relevant factors influencing your quality of life during the menopause transition is how you experience stressful life events. Everyone from every strata of life has stress come into her life in one form or another. Practicing the Transcendental Meditation technique does not mean that you are escaping from life's realities, but that you are using a tool that helps you handle stress without it overshadowing your life.

Picture it this way: Stress sometimes pours into your life like water pours into a bathtub until it overflows. Practicing the Transcendental Meditation technique is like pulling the plug from the tub. The water (stress) still flows in but it runs right out again. The TM technique pulls the plug on stress.

The Transcendental Meditation technique is the stress-handling technique I recommend because it works. It works not only for stress reduction but for so much more. It is a practical technology to increase success in daily life. Correct practice of this technique takes only 20 minutes practice twice a day, and involves no concentration or mental effort.

The Transcendental Meditation technique involves the use of sounds whose vibratory effect on the nervous system are especially beneficial. It is not a sound you have to concentrate on. Rather a sound is heard mentally. The sound is more like a vehicle that gets you to where you want to be.

The word "transcendental" means that during the Transcendental

LESS STRESS, LESS ANXIETY

Reduced Anxiety—Comparison of the *TM* Program with Relaxation Procedures

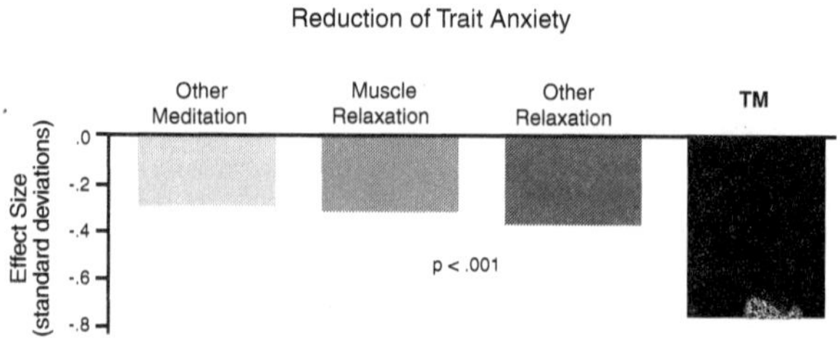

A statistical meta-analysis of all available studies (99 independent outcomes) indicated that the effect of the Transcendental Meditation program on reducing trait anxiety was approximately twice as great as that of all other meditation and relaxation techniques, including progressive muscle relaxation. Analysis showed that the positive result for the TM program could not be attributed to subject expectation, experimenter bias, or the quality of the research design.

This finding corroborates studies indicating that the TM technique produces substantially greater physiological effects than ordinary relaxation.

References: 1. K.R. Eppley, A.I. Abrams, and J. Shear, "Differential Effects of Relaxation Techniques on Trait Anxiety: A Meta-Analysis," *Journal of Clinical Psychology*, 45, (6) (1989). 2. M.C. Dillbeck, "The Effect of the Transcendental Meditation Technique on Anxiety Level," *Journal of Clinical Psychology*, 33 (1977), pp. 1076-1078.

Meditation technique the mind transcends, or goes beyond, even the subtlest impulses of the sound and other thought. The resulting experience is one of profound inner silence—with the mind wide awake, but still. This inner stillness is a field of unity and the source of thought.

Teachers of the TM technique are trained to choose these sounds to suit the individual. Just using any old sound or word doesn't work, because an appropriate sound for the most life-supporting effect is needed. A person also needs to understand the proper way of using the specific sound. After learning TM, the teacher makes sure that a student understands how to meditate properly and he or she answers questions concerning the new mental and physiological experiences of the new meditator. (See the Index for more information.)

I recommend the TM technique to my patients because it not only helps them reduce stress, it gives them a way to live the life they've always wanted to live. It helps with reducing stress, reducing free radicals, slowing down aging, and increasing success in daily life. More importantly, it can bring to the individual the optimum state of health known as enlightenment.

As Maharishi Mahesh Yogi, the founder of the TM program, has explained:

"It's only in the beginning days of meditation that one has to meditate in order to experience that silent, quiet level of the mind, that state of pure consciousness. As we continue to alternate the experience of meditation with daily activity, the value of that pure consciousness is infused into the mind. The pure level of consciousness becomes stabilized in our awareness. And when that pure level—the state of least excitation—is a living reality even during daily activity, this is the state of enlightenment. This is life free from suffering, life when every thought and action is spontaneously correct."[1]

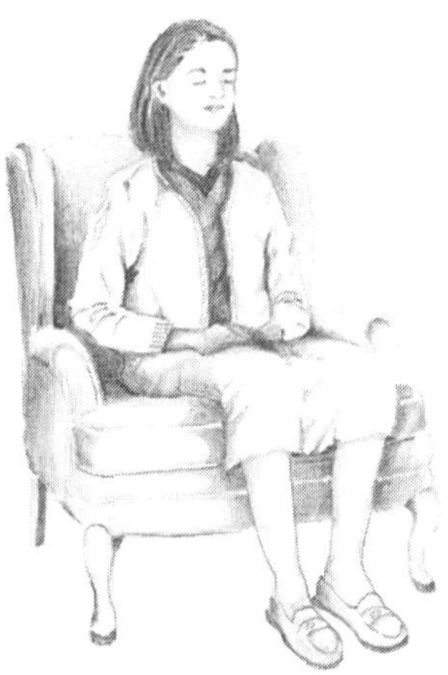

Practicing the *Transcendental Meditation* technique.

Research

More than 600 studies on the TM technique have been conducted at 210 universities and research centers in 30 countries around the world. The results have been published in more than 100 academic journals. Many doctors recommend the TM program to patients to reduce stress.

Dr. Kenneth Eppley, a researcher at Stanford Research Institute (SRI) International, has researched more than 100 meditation and relaxation techniques and found that they were

MORE RELAXED PHYSIOLOGY

Physiological Indicators of Deep Rest Through the *Transcendental Meditation* Technique

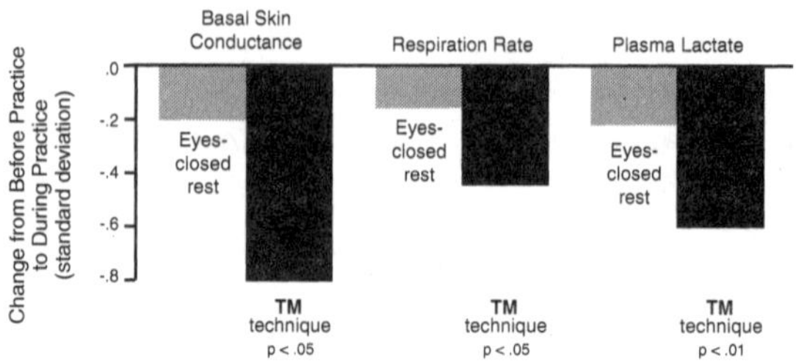

A meta-analysis found that the Transcendental Meditation technique produced a significant decrease in basal skin conductance compared to eyes-closed rest, indicating profound relaxation. Deep rest and relaxation were also indicated by similarly greater decreases in respiration rates and plasma lactate.

References: 1. M.C. Dillbeck and D.W. Orme-Johnson, "Physiological Differences between Transcendental Meditation and Rest," *American Psychologist*, 42 (1987), pp. 879-881.
2. R.K. Wallace, "Physiological Effects of Transcendental Meditation," *Science*, 167 (1970), pp. 1751-1754.
3. R.K. Wallace, et al., "A Wakeful Hypometabolic Physiologic State," *American Journal of Physiology*, 221 (1971), pp. 795-799.

not all equally effective. In the results of all the tests together, the Transcendental Meditation technique reduced anxiety more than twice as much as any other meditation or relaxation technique.[2]

People who practice the TM technique report feeling more alert and awake than usual. Studies have shown that the practice of TM generates an overall physiological rest and relaxation combined with an enriched blood supply to the brain.[3] Other research shows that during the practice of the TM technique, brain waves become more synchronized.[4] A deeper state of rest than just normal rest has also been found by practicing this technique. The autonomic nervous system becomes more stable during the practice of the TM technique than during eyes-closed rest.[5]

Free radical damage has been implicated in up to 80 percent of all human diseases, including atherosclerosis, cancer, heart disease, inflammatory diseases, degenerative diseases, and Alzheimer's.[6] Free radicals may cause much of the general deterioration of mind and body associated with aging.

One of the many known factors that generate excess free radicals is your body's reaction to stress. The fight-or-flight response to stress is built into your physiology to protect you from life-threatening situations. In our modern society, unhappy work relationships, children, partners, or having to deal with overwhelming situations can cause aggravations that lead to stress that you can't run from.

The body reacts to these stress-causing situations by generating cortisol and other stress-related chemicals that greatly increases free radical production. Since the body doesn't use this extra energy for fight or flight, it becomes like toxic waste to the body. The idea, then, would be to not let the physiology get so charged up at the sign of stress. Research shows that the TM technique, with its ability to counter stress, helps reduce free radical production.[7]

A number of studies have found that the TM technique helps to reverse or slow the aging process. One such study looked at DHEA-

Chronic Diseases Helped by the *Transcendental Meditation* Technique

Disorder	Per cent Improvement
Cardiovascular	92
Digestive tract	69
Musculoskeletal	94
Nose, throat, lung	89
Neurological	76
Glandular and metabolic	93
Mental health and substance abuse	92
Infectious disease	93
Skin disorder	86
Blood disorder	41

Reference: David W. Orme-Johnson, Ph D, and Robert E. Hernon, Ph D, "An Innovative Approach to Reducing Medical Care Utilization and Expenditures", *American Journal of Managed Care*, 1997, 3:135–144

DECREASED SUBTANCE ABUSE

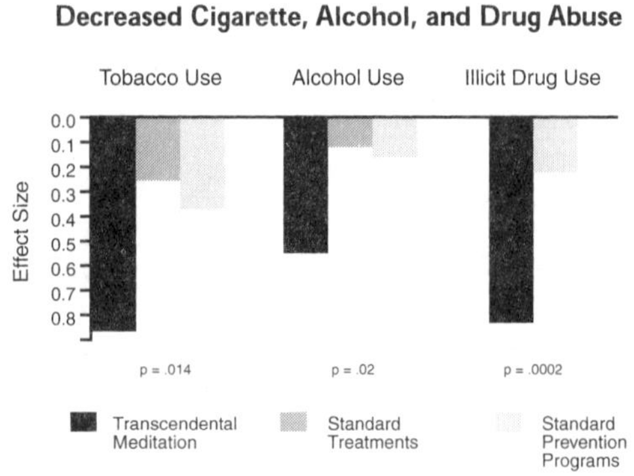

A statistical meta-analysis of 198 independent treatment outcomes found that the Transcendental Meditation program produced a significantly larger reduction in tobacco, alcohol, and illicit drug use than either standard substance abuse treatments (including counseling, pharmacological treatments, relaxation training, and Twelve-step programs) or prevention programs (such as programs to counteract peer-pressure and promote personal development). This meta-analysis controlled for strength of study design and included both heavy and casual users. Whereas the effects of conventional programs typically decrease sharply by 3 months, effects of Transcendental Meditation on total abstinence from tobacco, alcohol, and illicit drug ranged from 51%-89% over an extended time.

Reference: 1. "Treating and preventing alcohol, nicotine, and drug abuse through Transcendental Meditation: A review and statistical meta-analysis," *Alcoholism Treatment Quarterly*, vol. 11 (1994), pp. 13–87
2. "Effectiveness of the Transcendental Meditation program in preventing and treating substance misuse: A review," *International Journal of the Addictions* No. 26 (1991). pp. 293–325.

S. In a young adult, DHEA-S is the most abundant hormone in the body, but the levels decline rapidly with age. Women with high levels of DHEA-S are known to have less breast cancer and osteoporosis. It was found that people who practiced the TM technique had levels of DHEA-S that were as high as members of the control group who were five to ten years younger.[8]

The TM technique is also known to reduce substance abuse, such as alcohol, cigarettes and non-prescribed drugs.[9] Research on health insurance statistics and the health benefits of the TM technique showed that those who practiced the TM technique went to the hospital 56 percent less often for illness or surgery. The TM technique group needed 50 percent fewer doctors' visits.

This is a sampling of the scientific research that has been done on the TM technique. Research is ongoing around the world on the many benefits of this health-promoting technique.

A Fourth State of Consciousness

The distinct pattern of brain functioning found during the practice of Transcendental Meditation confirms Maharishi's description of the TM technique producing a fourth state of consciousness, Transcendental Consciousness, which is different from the three more familiar states of consciousness—waking, sleeping and dreaming.

The experience of Transcendental Consciousness involves what physics calls a field effect. It is thought that during the TM technique the mind is contacting a field that goes beyond the boundaries of the individual meditator's brain and spreads throughout a population. Thus, when a group practices the TM technique together, the environment also becomes more harmonious. Studies have shown that when individuals practice the TM technique and the advanced TM-Sidhi program in a group, it reduces crime and violence in the population as a whole.

The *TM-Sidhi* Program

The TM-Sidhi program trains the conscious mind to function in this field of pure consciousness. Maharishi Vedic Medicine maintains that this enriched experience balances all aspects of the physiology, and thereby prevents disease before it can happen.

More than 40 separate scientific studies show that when a sufficient percentage of the population practices the TM technique, or whenever a sufficient number of experts in the TM and TM-Sidhi programs practice their programs together, crime decreases, traffic accidents go down, and open warfare declines.[10]

COLLECTIVE HEALTH CARE

Maharishi Effect: Improved Quality of Life and Reduced Conflict in the Middle East Through Group Practice of the *Transcendental Meditation* and *TM-Sidhi* Programs

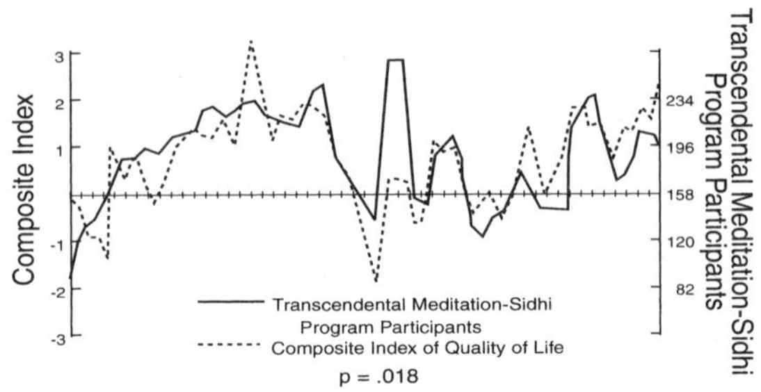

This study indicates that group practice of the Maharishi Transcendental Meditation and TM-Sidhi programs improved the quality of life in Israel as measured by improvements on an index consisting of reduced crime rate, reduced traffic accidents, reduced fires, the reduced number of war deaths in Lebanon, increases in the national stock market, and improvements in national mood. The chart above shows the strong correpondence between the number of TM-Sidhi program participants in the group in Jerusalem and a composite index of all the above variables.

References: 1. D.W. Orme-Johnson, C.N. Alexander, J.L. Davies, H.M. Chandler, and W.E. Larimore, "International Peace Project in the Middle East: The Effects of the Maharishi Technology of the Unified Field," *Journal of Conflict Resolution*, 32 (4) (1988), pp. 776-812.

2. J.L. Davies and C.N. Alexander, "Alleviating Political Violence Through Enhancing Coherence in Collective Consciousness: Impact Assessment Analyses of the Lebanon Wars," *Dissertation Abstracts International*, 49 (8) (1988), p. 2381A.

One of the ancient Vedic texts includes the phrase, "In the vicinity of the settled mind, hostile tendencies fall away." Just think of the positive consequences of that! Practicing the TM technique not only has a beneficial effect on your personal health, but when practiced in groups, can have a positive effect on the collective health of the world.

References

1. Oates, R.M., Jr. 1986. *Celebrating The Dawn.* Putnam. New York.
2. Eppley, K., Abrams, A., & Shear, J. 1989. Differential effects of relaxation techniques on trait anxiety: A meta-analysis. *Journal of Clinical Psych,* 45(6), 957–974.
3. Jevning, R., & Wilson A.F. 1978. Behavioral increase of cerebral blood flow. *The Physiologist,* 21, 60.
4. Levine, J.P. 1976. The Coherence Spectral Array and its application to the study of spatial ordering in the EEG. *Proceedings of the San Diego Biomedical Symposium,* 15, 237–247.
5. Dillbeck, M.C. & Orme-Johnson, D.W. 1987. Physiological differences between Transcendental Meditation and rest. *American Physiologist,* 42, 879–881.
6. Sharma, H. & Clark, C.1998 *Contemporary Ayurveda.* Philadelphia: Churchill Livingstone, p. 23.
7. Sharma, H.M. 1993 *Freedom From Disease.* Toronto. Veda Pubishing, 186–188.
8. Glaser, J.L., Brind, J.L., Vogelman, J.H. et al. 1992. Elevated serum dehydroepiandrosterone-sulfate levels in practitioners of the Transcendental Meditation (TM) and TM-Sidhi programs. *Journal of Behavioral Medicine,* 13(4), 327–341.
9. Alexander, C., Barnes, V., Schneider, R. et al. 1996. A randomized controlled trial of stress reduction on cardiovascular and all-cause mortality in the elderly: results of 8-year and 15-year follow ups. *Circulation,* 93(3) (abstract).
10. *Contemporary Ayurveda.* p. 147.

CHAPTER THREE

How Maharishi Vedic Medicine Looks at Menopause

Every woman experiences menopause differently. Phyllis came to me when she began to suffer from acute insomnia, which made her tired and "spacey" during the day. Her periods were highly irregular, coming every two weeks instead of every four weeks as usual. Phyllis was also suffering from many digestive problems, such as constipation, gas and bloating. Her skin was extremely dry, and Phyllis was sure she saw a new wrinkle appear every day.

Something peculiar was happening to Samantha, too. Samantha would wake up in the middle of the night sweating, sheets soaked, out of breath and frightened. Her reddish/auburn hair was turning prematurely gray, and she had frequent outbursts of intense, but irrational anger, which had begun to create problems in her marriage.

Margarite came to see me because of a sudden weight gain, which was of great concern to her, because she was already quite overweight. Her monthly periods had stopped altogether, and that made her happy because she had always had heavy monthly bleeding. However, other aspects of her life were making her miserable. She was feeling tired, lethargic and unhappy. She was starting to worry that this was the normal state of affairs for a woman in menopause.

Phyllis, Samantha and Margarite were all undergoing physiological changes associated with the transition into menopause. But they clearly experienced this process very differently. The reason for this is that each of them has a very different type of body. Each of us is born with a specific mind-body makeup, which profoundly influences all aspects of our being, from the structure of our physiology to our tastes, preferred activities and mental and emotional makeup. As we shall see in this chapter, the knowledge of the different mind-body makeup provides important insights into how your physiology might react during the transition into menopause. Understanding your own body type is also the first step in determining which health habits and natural treatments you should adopt to make this transition as smooth as possible.

The Three Doshas

Maharishi Vedic Medicine looks at two levels of symptoms of menopause—short-term and long-term. Short-term effects include hot flashes, vaginal dryness and mood swings. Long-term symptoms include osteoporosis and cardiovascular disease. To determine the cause of these symptoms, a physician trained in Maharishi Vedic Medicine examines the balance of the *doshas* in the body. The doshas are the three fundamental biological principles that control and regulate all physiological functions.

The concept of doshas provides important insights into the functioning of the physiology and the mechanics of enhancing well-being. The doshas should perhaps be referred to as mind-body constitutions, because they involve both physiological *and* psychological functions and characteristics. A person's Ayurvedic constitution is determined by the relative presence of the three doshas, Vata, Pitta, and Kapha. Each dosha regulates many functions in the mind-body system, but their functions can be summarized in three basic principles.

Vata controls any form of *movement* in the body, and as such is the dosha that governs transportation and communication in the body. Vata is involved in blood circulation, the passage of food through the digestive tract, breathing, and the movement of nerve impulses. Vata governs:

- The activity of the locomotor system
- Blood circulation
- The expansion and contraction of the lungs and heart

Vata is involved in intestinal peristalsis and elimination, activities of the nervous system, the contraction of the muscles, ionic transport across membranes, cell division, and unwinding of DNA during the process of transcription or replication. Here's how you can remember it: when wind or thoughts are moving, it's Vata that needs soothing.

Pitta governs *metabolism* and biochemical processes and it is responsible for the transformation of food, air and water into the building blocks of the physiology. Pitta rules the regions of the stomach and the small intestine. The energy processes Pitta governs are:

- The metabolic processes
- The enzymes which digest the food and extract energy—digestion and body heat
- The cells' energy-producing chemical reactions

If there is energy to be exchanged Pitta is at your service.

Kapha represents the principle of *structure*; it is the dosha that governs the formation of tissues, muscles, bones and sinews. Kapha gives solidity and balances the fluids. Kapha is responsible for:

- The structure and cohesion of organisms
- Biological strength
- Natural tissue resistance
- Proper body structure

Kapha influences the anatomical connections in the cell; it structures receptors and the various forms of chemical binding. Kapha can build anything.

The three doshas are responsible for the balance and healthy functioning of the physiology. Symptoms of ill health—including the problems associated with menopause result when the balance of one or more doshas is disturbed. When this happens, the functioning of one or several of the physiological activities that that dosha is responsible for will begin to be disrupted.

This marks the beginning of the disease process in the body. Disease does not emerge suddenly out of nowhere. It is the result of a gradual accumulation of imbalances in the body. When actual symptoms of disease become apparent, the person has reached one of the later stages in the gradual disruption of physiological functions, which we refer to as disease.

A range of behavioral, dietary, mental, emotional, and environmental factors can cause the doshas to go out of balance. The body is constantly acting and reacting to seasonal, dietary, lifestyle, emotional and mental patterns, and unless you know how to work with your specific body constitution, it is almost inevitable that imbalances will arise.

We all have all three doshas active in our physiology, but in varying combinations of predominance. If Vata dosha dominates in a person's physiology, for example, she will be a Vata body constitution, and both her mind and body will exhibit many of the characteristics associated with Vata. Because Vata is associated with the quality of air, lightness, and movement, such a person is typically thin and wiry, and she can eat copious amounts of food without ever gaining an ounce. Conversely, a person who is a pure Kapha constitution can barely look at food without the dial on the scale moving up. This is because Kapha is associated with the element of earth and has the qualities of density and heaviness.

Most people are not pure Vata, Pitta, or Kapha types. In many cases, people will have two or more predominant doshas, such as Vata/Pitta, Kapha/Vata, Pitta/Kapha, and so on.

All these elements which are active in your physiology are also active in your environment. They, in fact, are the same basic materials that make up everything in nature.

- Vata expresses itself in nature as *movement.*
- Pitta *transforms* something to something else.
- Kapha *builds* with it.

Once you understand them and the way they function, you will understand not only yourself, but why others act the way they do and why different seasons have different effects on your physiology.

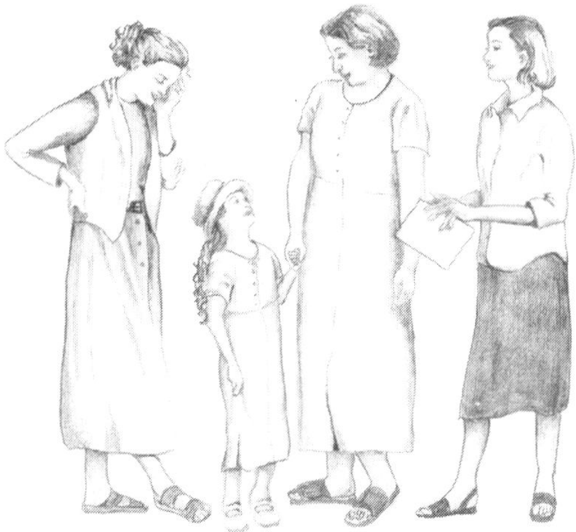

Most people's body types display a combination of the three doshas (Vata, Pitta, and Kapha) with one or two predominating.

A Look at Doshas in Balance and Out of Balance

Let's look at the doshas when they are in balance and when they are out of balance. Everyone has all three doshas active in her physiology in varying combinations of predominance. When the natural balance of the doshas is disturbed, ill health and problems associated with menopause can result.

A range of factors can cause this to happen. You may have created a Vata imbalance by irregular eating habits, eating rough, dry foods (such as crackers), rushing, mental overloading, or lack of adequate rest. Or a Pitta imbalance by too much sun, alcohol, too much focused mental work, visual strain, anger, or eating too much spicy, sour or salty food. A Kapha imbalance is created by lack of exercise, overeating, especially of heavy, oily, fat or sweet foods. A Kapha imbalance can be caused by lack of mental stimulation, or too much exposure to a damp, cold climate.

Vata Dosha

Remember Vata is associated with lightness, quickness, thinness, and also roughness and coldness. Women with a strong predominance of Vata are blessed with lightness and flexibility, charm and a sense of humor. In its healthy state Vata is expressed as joy, creativity and exuberance. Think of the thin, artistic, fun women you know who might also dance or practice yoga and you have a good picture of a Vata-type woman. Remember Vata is the "mover" so it is always on the go. In the physiology Vata "resides" regally in the head.

Because Vata is highly mobile and unstable, it is the most prone of the three doshas to be aggravated. When Vata is out of balance or there is too much Vata in a woman's physiology, Vata can manifest as unfounded fear, worry, insomnia and loneliness. A Vata type who is out of balance worries about everything, which makes her restless, sleepless, forgetful (always loses her keys, purse, etc.) and sometimes lonely for no reason.

In physiologies that are not so balanced, we see too much Vata expresses as dry skin, nails or nose, brittle bones, or forgetful memory. Dryness in the bowels results in constipation. Vata imbalance in the joints can cause certain types of arthritis. Out-of-balance Vata is also associated with conditions such as endometriosis, poor digestion and lightheadedness. A disturbance of Vata is present in all forms of premenstrual, menstrual, perimenopause and post-menopause problems.

Seasonally, Vata represents the windy season of late autumn and the cold season of winter. Vata Kala (*kala* means time) is the time of Vata influence. Menopause occurs in the Vata time of your life. In cultures where people are healthy and in balance Vata time can be exquisite. Qualities of wisdom and tranquility come into your life.

Menopause marks the time of your life when you move from being influenced by Pitta to being more influenced by Vata. Even if Vata did not dominate in your physiology before, signs of Vata's influence will show up at this time. Classic signs of increased Vata include thinner, drier skin and mucous membranes, thinning of the hair and bones, lighter sleep, and an increased tendency to worry. A key to eliminating any physiological or psychological discomfort associated with the transition into menopause is to balance the functioning of Vata dosha. Maharishi Vedic Medicine has many ways of avoiding these out-of-balance Vata symptoms through healthy eating habits (for your body type), specific herbs and proper daily routine.

Menopausal Symptoms Associated with Imbalanced Vata[1]

- Constipation or irritable bowel syndrome
- Dry skin or dry mucous membranes
- Insomnia
- Mood swings
- Reduced sex drive
- Worry

Pitta Dosha

The qualities associated with Pitta are heat, sour, slightly unctuous or oily, sharpness, pungency and fluidity. Women with a predominance of Pitta dosha tend to be intense, but the intensity, unlike Vata, is focused—more like laser light. This produces a sharp mind and clear, direct speech. Pitta types are decisive, efficient, and passionate. Pitta types are often courageous, clear-headed and successful.

Think of the women you know who are the achievers, the bosses, problem-solvers, dynamic and dramatic, and the ones who are on every committee because they can always be counted on to get the job done. The Pitta type is the one who thinks skydiving is fun. In the physiology, Pitta rules in the "gut." Feed this woman and she's happy.

In excess, Pitta can show up as a bad temper, heartburn, stress-associated heart attacks, peptic ulcers, colitis, acne, rashes, early graying and excessive hot flashes during menopause. An out-of-balance Pitta boss will scream at her staff, have skin break-outs, seem angry for no reason and will, in general, make people want to avoid her. She is the one in the women's room dashing cold water on her face due to hot flashes.

Seasonally, Pitta represents the hot season of summer and early autumn. Pitta Kala is the time in your life of Pitta influence. Pitta is the focused energy of the career-oriented adult. This time is when you are creating your career and family, setting and achieving goals and accomplishing many tasks. Perimenopause usually starts in the Pitta time of your life. Out-of-balance Pitta dosha plays a big part in menopausal symptoms. Because Pitta regulates hormonal balance, heat production and metabolism, it is the dosha primarily involved with hot flashes.

During the years of menstruation, impurities are eliminated each month with the menstrual flow. When this monthly cleansing stops, excess Pitta can build up. Maharishi Vedic Medicine can balance the Pitta dosha through introducing proper eating habits and herbal supplements that help calm a flare-up of Pitta. Soothing rejuvenation therapies from a Maharishi Ayur-Veda Health Center are also recommended. (See the Index for a list of Maharishi Ayur-Veda Health Centers.)

Menopausal Symptoms Associated with Imbalanced Pitta

- Excessive bleeding
- Hot flashes
- Irritability
- Skin irritations

Kapha Dosha

The qualities associated with Kapha are soft, cold, wet, unctuous, sweet, stable, shiny and heavy. Kapha creates strong bones and teeth, and the capability for storing energy, which may result in well-proportioned, heavier bodies. Kapha types often have big eyes, lustrous hair and inner calm. Kapha in its healthy state is unflappable, loyal, forgiving and sweet-spoken.

Women who have a predominance of Kapha are the original earth-mother or Venus types. They are the women who know about beauty and luxury, comfort and comfort food, who give loving and wise advice, whose houses can be full of kids and animals and still have room for more. These women will give you presents that you keep forever, handle problems in the office easily and with laughter. In general, Kapha rules the area of the heart.

Out-of-balance Kapha can give rise to congestion, sinus problems, asthma, diabetes and obesity or a tendency to gain weight. Kapha types can become complacent, lethargic, depressed and greedy. Often in our society we associate an out-of-balance Kapha with laziness, sloppiness and even stupidity. She has a hard time getting going in the morning, loves her sleep and "hides" from others. She gets depressed for not fitting in with society because of her weight, which makes her eat, which makes her more depressed.

Seasonally, Kapha is springtime when nature is rebuilding. With reference to stages in one's life, infancy is Kapha, the little chubby baby and childhood when young bodies are building.

Menopause and cardiovascular disease are often associated with each other, and out-of-balance Kapha types are susceptible to cardiovascular problems. Also depression is often associated with aging and menopause is associated with aging, too. But it shouldn't be—in many cultures menopause marks a woman's passage into wisdom.

Menopausal Symptoms Associated with Kapha

- Fluid retention
- High cholesterol or triglycerides
- Obesity
- Weight gain

If you lose touch with the inner intelligence of your body, you lose your natural sensitivity to your body and its needs. As a consequence, mistakes are made in your diet or daily routine and you end up eating foods or engaging in activities that disturb the functioning of the doshas. As a result, dosha imbalances gradually start to creep in.

The Doshas in Nature

The doshas operate in nature, too. Vata is movement, so it is represented by the wind and the motion of the water currents. Vata also represents cold, dryness, speed and lightness. Pitta is energy—sunshine and fire. Pitta also represents heat, sharpness and acidity. Kapha (the builder) is expressed in solid structures, such as rock and earth. Kapha shares Vata's quality of cold, and also represents heaviness, oiliness and slowness.

In nature you can really see the power of these three and what happens when one appears to be out of balance. They can cause havoc. Vata becomes a hurricane, Pitta is a heat wave, and Kapha drops an ice-cold blizzard on you. Think about what you would feel like if this happened in your physiology. Is not a hot flash just like an internal heat wave? Have you blasted someone like a hurricane or emotionally frozen someone out like a blizzard? Out-of-balance emotions, which can happen at menopause, can make you seem crazy. It causes your mate, children or grandchildren to tiptoe around the house, trying to be quiet because "Mom's gone mental" or menopausal. It's really the out-of-balance doshas.

If Vata is a nice windy day one moment and a hurricane the next, what is it like inside you? Vata, in charge of movement, can become out of balance through too much mental activity at night—thinking, worrying, thoughts scattered here and there, watching television shows (which are "moving" pictures and therefore Vata-aggravating)—and consequently cause insomnia. A common complaint from menopausal women is insomnia.

You already know what happens when Pitta turns up the heat—flash point. The heat can come out of your mouth in sharp words of anger. Ulcers and heartburn are also Pitta-related.

Kapha, when out of balance, can not only cause obesity, excessive sleep and depression, but can also cause cysts and other growths that women can experience at mid-life.

Linda, an American Indian, was having irregular periods at age 49 and felt cranky before and during her periods and was getting migraine headaches. She had cramps, lower back pain, digestive problems, pain and bloating, and chronic diarrhea or constipation. She told me she had irritable bowel syndrome and uncontrollable bowel movements to the point where it was debilitating and she was afraid to go anywhere. She also had endometriosis and ovarian cysts. She had been told that she had to have a hysterectomy which she didn't want to do.

Even though Linda was predominantly a Kapha/Pitta type of woman, it was obvious that all of her problems weren't simply Kaphic in nature. Since Vata is the lead dosha and will pull the other two doshas out of balance, Vata-balancing treatments are often recommended first.

I put Linda on a comprehensive program of the TM technique, dietary changes and specific herbal formulations, which addressed her problems, brought balance within the doshas and stabilized her hormones. Because the doshas involve both mind and body, their effects are both mental and physical. When they function normally they produce good health.

The three doshas are also represented by daily cycles, seasonal cycles, and even lifetime cycles. Remember, Vata Kala is the time of life from about age 50 on in which you become very wise and you can spread or move that wisdom around to help those not yet as wise as you.

The Mahabhutas

In Maharishi Vedic Medicine the doshas are considered to be among the first manifestations that appear as the primordial essence of life that transmutes into matter. The doshas are formed from combinations of the five basic elements, or the five *mahabhutas.* According to the ancient Vedic texts, the mahabhutas are five basic elements from which all of creation is derived. They are: space (sometimes translated as ether), air, fire, water and earth. Their Sanskrit names are: *akasha, vayu, tejas, jala* and *prithivi.*

Space and air equals Vata; fire and water equals Pitta; and earth and water equals Kapha. The mahabhutas are prior sproutings of consciousness into matter—prior to the doshas. They will be thoroughly discussed in a later chapter.

As for Linda and her perimenopausal problems, she said within the first month of learning the TM technique and following my recommendations, "I'm back to normal. I'm truly amazed—no diarrhea, no abdominal pain. I sleep through the night now and my weight is back to where it should be." The next month she said, "I have more energy, sleep through the night, my migraines have settled and I continue to have normal bowel movements with no cramping. I don't have up-and-down moods anymore. I feel happier and not so emotional."

References

1. Sharma, H. & Clark, C. 1998. *Contemporary Ayurveda.* Philadelphia: Churchill Livingstone, p. 37.

Chapter Four

Creating Balance

Women experience perimenopause and menopause differently depending on their body constitutions and how in balance the doshas are. Most women do not come to see me with only one obvious problem but with many. Sometimes they have been sent to one specialist after another because one antibiotic or other drug does not clear up all of their problems, yet all are related to an imbalance in the doshas.

For example Karla, a computer programmer, was perimenopausal with only three or four periods a year. She was experiencing breast tenderness and water retention, hot flashes, mood swings, lower back pain, lack of concentration, memory loss, sinus headaches and fatigue. She was also having chronic sinus problems.

In the area of digestion she was having chronic digestive problems, gas and bloating when eating most foods, irregular bowel movements and constipation. From time to time she would have diarrhea. She was told by her general practitioner that she had irritable bowel syndrome. She was also put on antibiotics for a month for the chronic sinus. When she came to me she also had a yeast infection, which was being treated. She had imbalances in Vata, Pitta and Kapha.

Everyone has to have all three doshas: Vata for motion, Pitta for energy and Kapha for structure, but the amounts differ in everyone. The balance of the doshas creates health, while imbalances in the doshas create the ground for disease. Therefore, to "balance the doshas" means to recreate the healthy and natural functioning of each dosha. To "balance the doshas" does not mean to create equal amounts of each dosha.

Most women are not purely Vata, Pitta or Kapha but usually have one or two doshas which predominate. Being a particular dosha type is not better than being another. Each woman's type of physiology is, or can be, perfect for her needs. I have seen many mind-body constitutions that are imbalanced. But when you see how perfect each person is when she is healthy and happy it doesn't matter what her mind-body makeup is. It's whether her constitution is healthy and balanced that matters.

In general, when you start to understand the three doshas, it becomes easy to identify when someone has a predominance of a particular dosha. This becomes very useful, not only in understanding yourself, but in understanding others and how to relate to them.

For example, let's take someone who is "the boss." If she is the Pitta type, she will have a clear intellect and make quick, clear decisions. If her Pitta is out-of-balance she will become angry and blame others for whatever has gone wrong. If you see anger expressed, you know it for what it is—an imbalance in the doshas. You don't lose sight of the wonderful woman she is deep inside. A woman with a predominance of Vata will also make quick, fair decisions; but if she is out-of-balance she will tend to blame herself for whatever has gone wrong. A Kapha-type of boss will be easy going with a very long fuse, and if something goes wrong, often she won't see the situation as being a problem. In these situations, too, you don't lose sight of the essential nature of each woman: you recognize that something has caused an imbalance and given rise to improper behavior of some sort.

You can look at children in the same way. Hot-headed, aggressive children tend to have a Pitta imbalance and will blame the world—hit out at it—for problems. A Vata type can have an attention deficit disorder—switching from one thing to another, always on the move. A Kapha child will have a tendency to overeat and might be withdrawn or depressed.

Women who are perimenopausal or into menopause can have these same problems. They can suddenly become angry, or forgetful or lethargic.

None of these problems has to happen. For a long, healthy life and worry-free menopause, Maharishi Vedic Medicine considers it essential that the doshas be kept in balance. This is accomplished by daily routine, by paying attention to daily cycles, and by taking rejuvenation and purification treatments at Maharishi Ayur-Veda Health Centers at least twice a year.

The Subdoshas

As you have learned, Vata is the dosha that is expressed in all motion in the physiology; Pitta is expressed in metabolism and Kapha rules over structure. According to the ancient Ayurvedic texts, each dosha has five subdivisions, called *subdoshas,* which have natural locations in the body where their influence is especially evident. It is as if each main dosha has five areas it "owns" and has sent the offspring to oversee them. There is one place where all three meet—the heart.

Disease often involves one or several of the subdoshas. Rheumatoid arthritis, for example, is linked to an imbalance in no less than five subdoshas: Vyana Vata, which is involved in circulation; Shleshaka Kapha, which is responsible for the lubrication of joints; Kledaka Kapha, which is associated with the functioning of the stomach; Pachaka Pitta, which is connected with the small intestine; and Samana Vata, which helps stimulate the digestive fluids.

Although you don't have to memorize the name of the subdoshas, it is important to have an understanding of their functions so that you have an understanding of what goes on inside your own physiology.

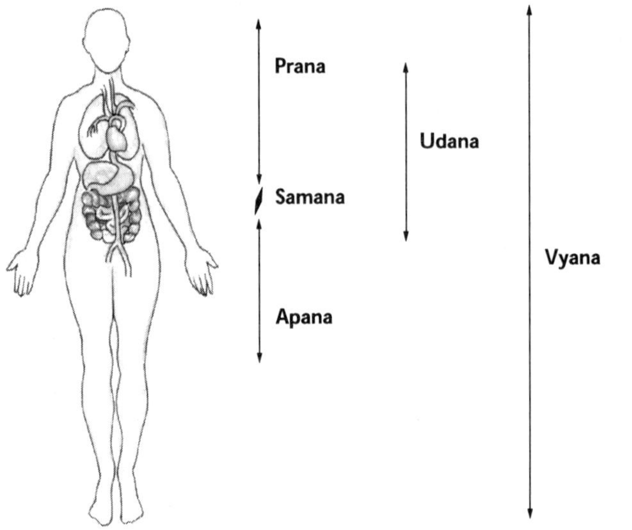

Locations of the five subdoshas of Vata.

The Five Subdoshas of Vata[1]

Vata's five subdoshas are called:
Prana Vata
Udana Vata
Samana Vata
Apana Vata
Vyana Vata

Prana Vata is located in the brain, head, throat, heart and respiratory organs. It is responsible for respiration, clarity of mind and reasoning, memory and enthusiasm. Prana Vata governs perception through all the senses, especially hearing and touch, and it recognizes feelings.

Out-of-balance Prana Vata can result in respiratory disorders, sneezing, belching, hiccups, memory problems, neurological disorders, tension headaches, worry, anxiety, overly active mind, insomnia, and asthma.

Just as Vata leads the doshas, Prana Vata leads the Vata

subdoshas—like the older child leads her siblings. Prana Vata is the most important subdosha to keep balanced as it is especially associated with the aging problems of memory loss, anxiety and insomnia.

Udana Vata is located in the navel, lungs and throat. It is responsible for the physiology of speech and singing. It governs energy, effort-making, strength and the act of swallowing.

Out-of-balance Udana Vata results in speech disorders, diseases of the throat such as soreness and dry coughs, and fatigue.

Samana Vata is located in the stomach and the intestines. It is responsible for peristaltic motion and for cooling the Pitta which digests food.

Out-of-balance Samana Vata results in weak or irregular digestion, bloating and anorexia.

Apana Vata is located in the colon, bladder, navel, thighs, groin, sexual organs and rectum. Its responsibilities are: the elimination of wastes, sexual discharge and menstruation. The location of Apana Vata in the colon is considered the principle seat of Vata.

Imbalanced Apana Vata results in: constipation, diarrhea, flatulence, colitis, lower back pain and back spasms, sexual dysfunctions, and menstrual problems.

Vyana Vata is spread throughout the body in the skin, nervous system, and circulatory system. Its functions are: circulation, blood pressure, and the sense of touch.

Conditions resulting from out-of-balance Vyana Vata are: circulatory and heart diseases (such as high blood pressure and heart arrhythmia) and nervous diseases.

In order to understand and eliminate any "abnormalities" caused by menopause, it is important to understand that the conditions ascribed to menopause (such as forgetfulness, dizziness, headaches, constipation, insomnia, worry and depression) are mostly signs that Vata dosha and/or Vata subdoshas are out of balance. Remember, even if Vata is not your primary constitution,

Vata dosha is the first dosha to go out of balance and, therefore, is the dosha that should receive the most attention. When Vata dosha is back in balance then it tends to draw the other doshas back in balance with it.

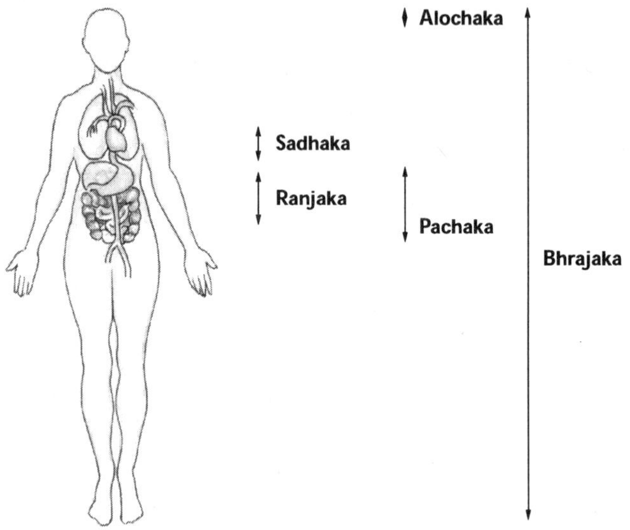

Locations of the five subdoshas of Pitta.

The Five Subdoshas of Pitta

Women with a predominance of Pitta dosha are susceptible to stomach disorders of a Pitta nature—the high-powered woman who gets an ulcer is the perfect example of an imbalance in Pitta. Pitta imbalances can show up at the time of menopause as hot flashes, night sweats, skin rashes, irritability, heartburn and visual problems.

The five subdoshas of Pitta are:

Pachaka Pitta
Ranjaka Pitta
Sadhaka Pitta
Alochaka Pitta
Bhrajaka Pitta

Pachaka Pitta is located in the stomach and small intestines and is responsible for the digestion of food and the separation of waste products.

Imbalanced Pachaka Pitta results in weak digestion, heartburn, ulcers and hyperacidity.

Ranjaka Pitta is located in the liver, spleen, duodenum and red blood cells. Ranjaka, which is a Sanskrit word meaning "to color," is responsible for the formation of red blood cells. It balances the blood chemistry. Toxins in the physiology greatly disturb Ranjaka Pitta.

When Ranjaka Pitta becomes out of balance the results can be anemia, blood disorders, skin problems, jaundice, anger and hostility.

Sadhaka Pitta is located in the heart and, therefore, governs the emotions and contentment. It is very interesting to note that Sadhaka Pitta also governs memory and intelligence. The phrase "think with your heart, not your head" has great significance when you realize that memory and intelligence is the concern of Sadhaka Pitta, which resides in the heart area.

Depression and related conditions are the result of imbalanced Sadhaka Pitta. Heart disease, memory loss and indecisiveness are also governed by Sadhaka Pitta.

Alochaka Pitta is located in the eyes; therefore, it governs eyesight. Sharp, clear eyesight is the concern of Alochaka Pitta, while all visual problems, including bloodshot eyes, are the sign of imbalance in that subdosha.

Bhrajaka Pitta is located in the skin and is in charge of skin metabolism. An imbalance of Bhrajaka Pitta arises as skin disorders, especially those of a fiery Pitta nature such as rashes, acne and boils.

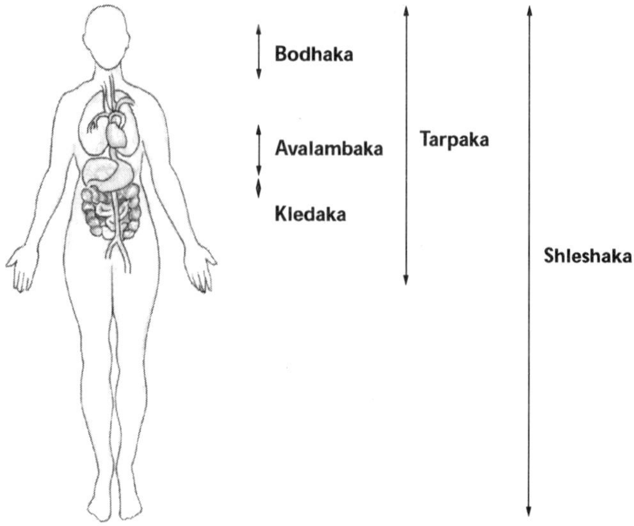

Locations of the five subdoshas of Kapha.

The Five Subdoshas of Kapha

Weight gain and other dietary changes can occur at this time of a woman's life due to Kapha dosha and its subdivisions. A feeling of lethargy and joint problems are also governed by the Kapha subdoshas.

The subdoshas of Kapha are:

Kledaka Kapha
Avalambaka Kapha
Bodhaka Kapha
Tarpaka Kapha
Shleshaka Kapha

Kledaka Kapha is located in the stomach. Its function is the moistening and initial digestion of food. If Kledaka Kapha is out of balance then all the other Kapha subdoshas will be adversely affected. An imbalance in this subdosha manifests itself as dull digestion. It is important to understand Kledaka Kapha because, in Maharishi Vedic Medicine, a strong digestion is the key to good health.

Avalambaka Kapha is located in the chest, heart, lungs and lumbar regions. Avalambaka Kapha supports the heart and lumbar region and gives strength and stamina in these areas.

An imbalance in Avalambaka Kapha results in back pain, heart problems, asthma, wheezing, chest congestion and lethargy.

Bodhaka Kapha is located in the area of the tongue and throat. It is in charge of the perception of taste, the moistening of the tongue, and the secretion of mucus in the mouth.

If Bodhaka Kapha is out of balance the perception of taste can become distorted along with salivation. Diseases may arise in the oral cavity and tongue.

Tarpaka Kapha is located in the head, sinuses and cerebrospinal fluid. The function of Tarpaka Kapha is the moistening in the nose, mouth and eyes; maintaining spinal fluid; and nourishment of the mind and the sense and motor organs.

Sinus problems, nasal congestion, sinus headaches, problems with the sense of smell as well as the other senses, and coughing which originates from the upper respiratory tract, are all related to an imbalance of Tarpaka Kapha subdosha.

Shleshaka Kapha is located in the joints. Shleshaka Kapha is in charge of lubrication of joints throughout the body. It is also in charge of cohesion and binding.

Problems with the joints are due to an imbalance in Shleshaka Kapha's domain.

As you can see from learning about the subdoshas, your own physiology will have several areas that need to be brought back into balance for a smooth transition into the next half of your life.

Everything in Working Order

Pitta takes things in, Vata moves it, and Kapha builds with it. All of the doshas and subdoshas have to be functioning together in a balanced way for the mind and physiology to be healthy.

But, if even one subdosha is not functioning in balance then everything in your life can seem out of whack. If Sadhaka Pitta (which governs the emotions) is blocked, then it can have an effect on chemicals that are necessary for proper brain functioning. For example, when Sadhaka Pitta is out of balance, it leads to anger—especially against a loved one: "OH, YOU, you're no good. You did this, this and this to me. Why don't you do this and act like so-and-so?"

Or it leads to anxiety—"I couldn't sleep because of all this stuff you told me last night, so here I am waking you up at 3:30 a.m. so we can discuss it now and I can get some sleep afterwards." Or to insecurity: "I need reassurance that you still love me every day; why don't you talk to me more, or call me from work, or invite me to lunch, or hug and kiss me more often?"

And particularly during menopause, or perimenopause, with Pitta and Vata playing a duel over who gets control, you have a recipe for one impossible person to get along with. "I don't want to do any more fun stuff with you, until you're ready to sit down and talk and process your feelings!" The poor person at the other end of this nonsense has no idea what "process your feelings" even means.

By diagnosing the dosha imbalances underlying a specific disease, a physician trained in Maharishi Vedic Medicine often is able to address problems that don't respond to the therapies of Western medicine.

As for Karla and her multitude of problems—her imbalanced Vata was causing lower back pain, memory loss and lack of concentration. Oil self-massage, good sleep habits, and the TM technique are major factors in helping to put Vata back into balance. After looking into her eating habits I placed her on a Kapha-pacifying diet for her chronic sinus problems, water retention, yeast infection and depression. Special herbal recommendations and calming yoga stretches helped with her Pitta problems.

In less than a month she reported that she was doing much better—less post nasal drip, fewer headaches and hot flashes, less tired. She wasn't feeling moody or depressed anymore. The yeast infection had cleared up and she was having daily bowel movements. Karla told me, "I cannot believe that I could get better so quickly as I have been suffering with these various problems for years."

As with all my patients I reminded Karla that conventional medicine is for crisis management but Maharishi Ayur-Veda is for every day. A month of Maharishi Ayur-Veda will make you better. A year of Maharishi Ayur-Veda will transform your life at all levels—physical, mental, emotional and spiritual. Karla followed my advice and transformed herself.

References

1. Sharma, H. & Clark, C. 1998. *Contemporary Ayurveda.* Philadelphia: Churchill Livingstone, pp. 40–41.

CHAPTER FIVE

Long-Term Influences on Menopausal Health

As you have probably figured out by now, most people are not purely Vata, Pitta, or Kapha. While everyone's mind-body constitution has a predominance of one or two doshas, it is usually a mixture such as Vata/Pitta. As you already know, everyone has all three doshas. When each dosha is functioning properly, it is considered balanced: Balancing the doshas, therefore, does not mean that each dosha is equal to each other, but that they are balanced within themselves. People with a predominance of a certain dosha are more likely to develop diseases related to that dosha.

The Ten Types of Doshas

The three doshas of Vata, Pitta and Kapha combine to make 10 different constitutions.

1. Vata	2. Pitta	3. Kapha
4. Vata/Pitta	5. Vata/Kapha	6. Pitta/Vata
7. Pitta/Kapha	8. Kapha/Vata	9. Kapha/Pitta
10. Vata/Pitta/Kapha		

Vata

Physically, Vata women are thin, with thin arms and legs, have little fat and do not gain weight easily. They can be either tall or short. Their hair and skin are dry. Their immune systems might be weak or variable.

When in balance a Vata woman has a high degree of intuition and inspiration. She can be social, very active, but not necessarily gregarious. She likes to move and travel. She is bubbly and full of joy.

When a Vata woman is out of balance, she will worry, be anxious, fearful and nervous. Vaginal dryness is caused by an imbalance of Vata. Fatigue, pain and cramping are part of her menses.

Pitta

Physically, a Pitta-type woman can have a fair or reddish complexion and will sunburn easily. She can be shapely, but usually can keep the weight under control. She can be prone to dandruff, or have slightly oily hair, which may gray prematurely. She has to watch out for vaginal or urinary infections.

When in balance the Pitta woman is highly dynamic and motivated. She is determined, intelligent, discriminating, passionate and knowledgeable on many subjects, making her a natural leader and teacher.

When out of balance the normally dynamic Pitta woman becomes angry, frustrated, manipulative and jealous. Her body heats up which brings inflammation to the body, mind and spirit. If she is still experiencing her monthly cycle, she will display symptoms of premenstrual syndrome (PMS).

Kapha

Physically, a Kapha woman is larger than her Vata and Pitta sisters. She has bigger bones and is just more physically big and strong in general. If she gets proper exercise, she can be healthy looking with a "normal" weight or be overweight. She tends to have beautiful hair and skin. She often has poor circulation making her prone to cellulite. Since a Kapha woman has a strong immune system and good stamina, she tends to be healthy.

When in balance the Kapha woman is very nurturing and stable, both mentally and emotionally. She is the real "earth mother" and those who need that stability in their lives will naturally gravitate to her. She can be considered Venus incarnate. When in balance a woman who is predominantly Kapha will be self-oriented and reliable—not too much bothers this woman. She is often surrounded by abundance.

When out of balance she will be overweight and lethargic and she will feel insecure, unloved and needy. She has a tendency to accumulate water in the physiology. She can lose her natural luster and look drawn-out and tired. This is the one type that needs to exercise more than the others. However, she doesn't like to, unless she makes it a positive addiction in her life.

Vata/Pitta

These women are less thin than the purely Vata type, with more strength and muscles, which are the added Pitta qualities. They have more stamina and focused intellects, can tolerate cold a little better, and are more enthusiastic. Their hair may be thin and dry if they favor Vata, or oily with dandruff if they favor Pitta, or a combination of both. They can be thin with pimply complexions. Menstruation is irregular.

When in balance the Vata/Pitta combines the qualities of quickness with dynamism and can be very creative and successful in any direction she puts her mind to. Vata/Pitta types make good teachers with lots of energy and lightness of spirit.

A Vata/Pitta woman who is out of balance can become erratic emotionally, which leads to emotional and impassioned outbursts. Inflammations or infections can be common. Vaginal dryness can also be common.

Donna has the slight yet strong build and active personality of a Vata/Pitta type. She told me that when her menses stopped she seemed to have a personality change that caused her and her family great concern. When she came to see me she was worried that she was going slightly crazy and that it was all due to menopause.

She said in a rush that this was not how she wanted to live the rest of her life and to please do something. From the way she spoke and from the list of her complaints, it was easy to see that her Vata had become imbalanced and her Pitta followed suit. She had switched from being bubbly to being anxious and she feared the worst (but was vague as to what that was).

Her complaints were lower back pain, and pain in her right arm especially in the elbow region (which had been investigated and no cause had been found). She was also experiencing stiffness and pain in the neck, and some numbness and tingling in her hands and feet. She had been to chiropractors and acupuncturists, which had given her some relief but did not take away her discomfort. Typically, because Vata was out of hand, she was having sleep problems.

Rosa has the same type of physiology as Donna, Vata/Pitta, yet she was having more Pitta-type problems: hot flashes, acid stomach, and anger bordering on rage. She was also a sun worshiper and spent as much time as possible exercising, especially jogging, in the sun. Although Rosa has always had a "feisty" personality, when she started experiencing perimenopause her feistiness turned to fire. Her highly spiced diet had to be toned down and her body cooled down in order for her to feel better, which were not the original recommendations made to Donna.

Although these two women have the same body type, their problems were almost entirely different and had to be treated differently—a concept which Western medicine does not seem to understand.

Vata/Kapha

A Vata/Kapha woman can be either thin and wiry, or she can have a Kapha-type body that allows her to have more defined muscles in her arms and legs. The Kapha may make her more slow-moving. These women tend to have poor circulation with cold hands and feet and don't like the cold weather in general. If she is thin with oily skin, then she is likely to be a Vata/Kapha type.

Vata/Kapha women in balance have excellent intuition. They gravitate towards people and animals and love nature. They have the earthy qualities of Kapha with the mental intuition of Vata. They can be quick and efficient or calm and relaxed.

Lack of balance in this mind-body constitution causes feelings of worthlessness, guilt, depression and rejection. Digestion is slow or irregular. She may have joint pain, sinus problems and excess mucus.

Pitta/Vata

This woman is a little stronger and more muscular than the thinner Vata type. But she still may be lean. She has oilier skin and hair than the Vata/Pitta type. She will burn more easily in the sun and may break out in pimples.

In balance she is very quick-moving, friendly and talkative combined with the focused intellect, energy, and stamina of the Pitta constitution. Generally she is passionate about her interests. She will also have a stronger digestion and more regular elimination. She can tolerate cold better than a pure Vata woman. The Pitta/Vata woman is an enthusiastic problem solver.

The Pitta/Vata woman who is out of balance can become angry, which comes out of her mouth in violent outbursts of blame towards others. Her emotions are up and down. Out-of-balance Pitta/Vata constitutions have to be careful of infections in the vagina or bladder.

Pitta/Kapha

Physically, she is more muscular than the Pitta/Vata—solid and sturdy instead of wiry and thin. She has what is considered an athletic build and has the advantage of the energy of Pitta and the stamina of Kapha.

These women have a combination of the dynamism and sharp intellect of Pitta along with the stability of Kapha. She can be the career woman who manages her household very well too. She has the capacity to work. Her circulation is good.

A Pitta/Kapha who is imbalanced is a workaholic who can feel frustrated and angry if things are not going fast enough for her. She will hold in her emotions until they burst out of her mouth in inappropriate language. She has to watch out for yeast infections.

Kapha/Vata

Physically, a Kapha/Vata woman is larger than the Pitta/Vata or Vata/Pitta combinations. Her skin and hair are good due to the combination of oiliness of Kapha and the dryness of Vata.

When in balance this woman is very friendly and social. She takes both the goodness and stability of Kapha along with the lightness of Vata. She can have loads of stamina, listens to others and is a good manager and care giver.

When out of balance she has feelings of unworthiness, depression, feels unloved and unhappy. She internalizes these feelings and seldom lets them out as a Pitta woman would. Her skin may be dry.

Kapha/Pitta

Physically, she is a bigger woman who is very fit and strong. If she exercises properly she can create a powerful body.

When in balance she is strong, powerful and can basically do whatever she wants in life. She has a good disposition and tends to help the "underdog" or less fortunate person.

When out of balance she can hold in her anger just so long and then, watch out—she aims it at all around her. She has a tendency to accumulate water which makes her feel uncomfortable and bloated. She also is susceptible to yeast infections.

Vata/Pitta/Kapha

This tri-dosha combination—called *samadoshas*—combines all three of the characteristics of Vata, Pitta and Kapha. This type of woman is said to be rare and she will have perfect balance of all three doshas. A woman with this type of constitution is less likely to become imbalanced than all the other types. She will have tremendous flexibility and stability.

When she is in balance she has all the greatest qualities of a beautiful woman—love, strength of character, intuition, and willpower.

Of course, when this woman is out of balance, she can have the problems of all three of the doshas. Since Vata leads the other two doshas, she will show this imbalance first. An imbalance of Pitta will cause anger and breakouts while Kapha will cause congestion and internalized emotions.

Your Balanced Nature at Birth—Prakriti
Your Current Imbalance—Vikriti

When you are born you have a certain constitutional type—a basic nature. You can see this in little babies—small and thin with a predominance of Vata; big heavy babies with a predominance of Kapha; medium-sized babies might have a predominance of Pitta. It's not always obvious. This natal constitution is called in Sanskrit the *janma prakriti.* The janma prakriti is the constitution you were born with and may change gradually over a lifetime, to what is known as the *deha prakriti.*[1]

There is also a changing nature in the physiology called the *vikriti.* For example, a cold is a transient imbalanced state in the physiology, but it doesn't indicate a change in your basic nature or prakriti. While your constitution is always changing (vikriti), your basic constitution is always the same (prakriti). When your changing constitution is the same as your natal constitution, then you are considered healthy.

For example, suppose you were born with a Vata-type nature which would be your prakriti, but your Pitta dosha becomes imbalanced. You would appear to be a Pitta type. But after treatment by a physician skilled in Maharishi Ayur-Veda, you would become balanced and your true Vata nature of lightness and brightness would appear. The fiery qualities of imbalanced Pitta would simply disappear.

The Seven Dhatus

Many of the short-term problems associated with menopause can be addressed by simply balancing the three doshas. The long-term problems that often emerge after the onset of menopause, however, are linked to deeper physiological imbalances on the level of the bodily tissues, or *dhatus.* Dysfunction at the level of the dhatus represents a more advanced stage of the disease process, because at this point, imbalances in the doshas have migrated to the body tissues, causing disruption and disease. Osteoporosis, for example, is associated with a malfunctioning in the formation of the bone tissue.

The bodily tissues, or dhatus, play an important role in maintaining health and preventing disease. Any disturbance in the equilibrium of the dhatus will manifest as some form of disease—osteoporosis, cardiovascular disease, cancer—or any of the other serious health concerns that are associated with aging. The combination of imbalanced doshas and abnormal dhatus is one of the most decisive developments in the gradual breakdown of the body's natural equilibrium. Once physiological imbalances reach this level, it is much harder to reverse the disease process. This is why Maharishi Vedic Medicine places such great emphasis on eliminating imbalances in the body long before they show up as disturbances in the tissues. To understand how you can prevent the long-term problems associated with menopause, it is necessary to understand the nature of the bodily tissues and how they develop.

The progression of doshic imbalances becoming full-fledged disease is usually a gradual and slow process. Disease develops through the gradual accumulation of aggravated or excess doshas, and the excess dosha energy can circulate in the body tissues for quite a while before developing into disease. If the imbalance is mild and the natural strength of the body is strong, then the inherent self-regulating intelligence of the body can usually correct the imbalance and halt the progression of disease. If the imbalance is moderate or severe, however, therapeutic measures need to be applied to prevent it from causing disruption to the bodily tissues.

The seven dhatus develop in the following sequence:

1. Rasa dhatu: the principle upholding the first products of digested food. It is responsible for blood plasma and lymph fluids.
2. Rakta dhatu: the principle upholding blood. It is responsible for hemoglobin, the oxygen-carrying component.
3. Mamsa dhatu: muscle.
4. Meda dhatu: fat and connective tissue.
5. Asthi dhatu: bone.
6. Majja dhatu: bone marrow and the central nervous system.
7. Shukra dhatu: ova and sperm.

Each tissue level is constantly reformed and nourished on a daily basis. Therefore, a balanced rakta level can only be created from a fully developed and balanced rasa level, on down the line. Impurities within one level of tissue can interfere with the ability to create balanced tissues at the next level.

For example, women with meda (responsible for fat) out of balance will be more prone to obesity, diabetes and cardiovascular disease. And if meda is out of balance, the next level, asthi (responsible for bone), becomes improperly nourished. As a result, the bones become weak, as in osteoporosis; and hair, nails and teeth are negatively affected. Therefore, many of the symptoms of menopause are interrelated through the functioning and formation of the tissues.

If the dhatus are functioning properly, then they reveal these signs of health. Note that these signs show up a great deal on the skin. The skin, then, is a mirror to the health of your physiology.

What the seven healthy dhatus show:

1. Rasa: unctuous and smooth, soft lustrous skin; clear, fine, deep-rooted hair.
2. Rakta: unctuous and ruddy face.
3. Mamsa: stable, large, well-formed musculature.
4. Meda: oily complexion; healthy plumpness but not obese.
5. Asthi: well-formed bones and joints.
6. Majja: softness of organs; long, rounded joints.
7. Shukra: gentle look, milky whites of eyes, clear and unctuous complexion.

Since level one, rasa, is concerned with the first products of digestion, it is disrupted by overeating, especially of the harder to digest cold, heavy or oily foods. Too much mental activity can disrupt rasa, too. The brain is digesting too much information.

Level two, rakta, is disrupted by too much exposure to the heat and sun, and overly hot foods and drinks.

Mamsa is disrupted by overly heavy or bulky foods.

Meda is aggravated by lack of exercise, sleeping too much in the day, fatty food, and alcohol.

Asthi is aggravated by too much exercise, excessive jerking movements, and constant use of Vata-aggravating food and behavior.

Majja is disrupted by certain toxic substances and crushing bone injuries.

Shukra is aggravated by too much sexual indulgence.

The traditional rejuvenation treatments of Maharishi Ayur-Veda are especially effective in balancing the transformation of the tissues. When the tissues are balanced before and at the onset of menopause, symptoms of imbalanced tissues, such as cardiovascular disease and osteoporosis, should not appear.

How the Dhatus Develop Sequentially to Form Shukra Tissue

rasa ▶ rakta ▶ mamsa ▶ meda ▶ ashti ▶ majja ▶ shukra

DHATUS	CORRESPONDING TISSUES
Rasa	plasma, the first product of digestion and metabolism
Rakta	blood, including hemoglobin
Mamsa	muscle tissue
Meda	fat tissue
Asthi	bone tissue
Majja	bone marrow, tissue of the nervous system
Shukra	reproductive tissues

Ojas

All the dhatus arise from a biochemical substance known in Maharishi Vedic Medicine as *ojas,* which pervades the physiology. Ojas is the essence of all the dhatus. It is the holistic value, the finest material value of the dhatus and the finest material end product of digestion.

According to the ancient Ayurvedic texts, when the quality of ojas is lessened too much, life itself is threatened. Ojas is the substance considered to connect consciousness with matter. Between one dhatu and the next a specific type of ojas is formed, out of which the next dhatu is created. The type of ojas formed is different in each one of these stages. Therefore, there are eight types of ojas. One type at the beginning of rasa dhatu, one between each dhatu, and one at the end of shukra dhatu.

The sequential development of the dhatus

ojas ▶ rasa ▶ rakta ▶ mamsa ▶ meda ▶ ashti ▶ majja ▶ shukra ▶ ojas

⬍ ⬍ ⬍ ⬍ ⬍ ⬍

ojas ojas ojas ojas ojas ojas

How to develop healthy ojas in the physiology is discussed in the chapter on diet and digestion.

The Thirteen Agnis and Their Functions

One of the main branches of Ayurvedic treatment is called *kayachikitsa*, or "therapy of fire." *Kaya* means "fire" and *chikitsa* "therapy of." Kayachikitsa is all about maintaining and balancing the digestive fire, *agni*. As you learned earlier, the body is made up of the five basic elements, one of which is fire. In the human body, this fire or heat takes the form of the digestive liquids, known as agni in the ancient Ayurvedic texts. Agni has the qualities of heat and transformation, just as a flame of a fire.

There are thirteen different forms or qualities of agni, each of which play a certain role in transforming food into the bodily tissues—blood, bones, fat, and skin. The main location of agni is the digestive juices in the large and small intestines and the stomach. This is called the *jatharagni*, which is responsible for transforming the food we eat into the nutrient plasma that circulates throughout the body and nourishes all the cells and tissues. Even though all of the five elements form the jatharagni, it is mainly fire. And even though it is liquid, it does not have the cold, moist qualities of liquid. Rather it is like a cooking fire, and is responsible for cooking or digesting the food.

The jatharagni is made up of five *bhutagnis*. They represent each of the five elements, and help to digest food made up of the corresponding element. For example, *prithivi agni* (related to prithivi, or earth) helps break down food of a more heavy, solid, earthy constituency, *apagni* (related to apa, or water) helps break down watery foods, and *tejasagni* (related to tejas, or fire) helps break down spicy or hot foods.

Seven Dhatu Agnis

There are also seven agnis for the seven dhatus (tissues) of the body, which transform one tissue into the other in the process of digestion. Each dhatu agni has a very specific task to transform the previous dhatu into the next dhatu in the sequence.

The agnis that relate to the seven dhatus, are called the seven dhatu agnis:

- Rasa agni
- Rakta agni
- Mamsa agni
- Meda agni
- Asthi agni
- Majja agni
- Shukra agni

The thirteen agnis work in a sequence to digest the food you eat. When you eat a carrot, the jatharagni "cooks" or transforms the food into two substances, the *rasa* (essence of food) and the *mala* (waste products) of food. These two substances go through further transformations when digested by the five bhutagnis, and then get converted into rasa dhatu, the first tissue of the body.

Once you understand the role agni plays in nourishing the dhatus, you can see why maintaining the digestive fire is essential for health. For example, a disturbance in meda agni—which is located in the dhatu concerned with body fat—may cause you to gain too much weight. A disturbance in rakta agni could cause a blood disorder.

How Imbalanced Jatharagni Leads to Disease

The strength of the dhatu agnis depends on the strength of the jatharagni. If the jatharagni is strong and in balance, then the dhatu agnis will be strong and in balance. That is why a strong digestion is central to good health according to Maharishi Vedic Medicine.

A balanced jatharagni produces the clear, thin, odorless, unctuous nutrient fluid, called rasa dhatu. Rasa dhatu is the first product of digested food, and when it is properly digested, it nourishes all of the other dhatus and is capable of entering the smallest pores of the body to provide nutrition to the tiniest cell.

When jatharagni is out of balance, it does not break down the food properly and creates unhealthy or unusable nutrient materials. For example, if agni is too strong it burns or chars the food, as if you burned the food on your stove. Weak or dull agni produces undigested or inadequately digested food, and erratic agni produces a mixture of digested and undigested food.

Factors that Derange Agni[2]

- Fasting
- Overeating
- Irregular eating
- Eating before previous meal is digested
- Eating during indigestion
- Unwholesome food
- Suppression of natural urges
- Faulty adaptation of place, climate, season
- Emotions such as anger, worries, sorrow

The Malas

The malas are the body's waste products. They are formed as a by-product of the work of the agnis in metabolizing and transforming food and the dhatus. The malas contain all five mahabhutas (space, air, fire, water, earth), and each is related to a specific dhatu. Each dhatu has related malas. For example:

Rasa dhatu, which is responsible for plasma and lymph fluids, has as its waste material, mucus.

Rakta dhatu, which is responsible for blood, has as its waste material, digestive bile.

Mamsa dhatu, which is responsible for muscle, has as its waste material, excreta from outer orifices—e.g., ear wax.

Meda dhatu, which is responsible for fat and connective tissue, has as its waste material, sweat.

Ashti dhatu, which is responsible for bones, has as its waste material, nails and hair.

Majja dhatu, which is responsible for marrow and nerves, has as its waste material, tears.

Shukra dhatu, which is responsible for ova and sperm, has as its waste material, smegma.

The Thirteen Srotas

The srotas are thirteen channels of circulation that carry both subtle and gross matter in the body. They move and nourish the seven dhatus and they also nourish the organs and help to eliminate the waste products (malas) from the body. These clear channels are an indicator of good health.

The srotas can be disrupted in four ways: obstruction, excessive flow, diverted flow, and structural changes. Atherosclerosis, the thickening of blood vessel walls that leads to stiffness, brittleness, and narrowing of the passageway, is a primary example of obstruction. Dysentery is an excessive flow through the srotas; diverted flow is the improper shunting of blood; and one example of structural changes can be seen in the atheroma that develops in atherosclerosis.

An imbalance in the doshas can aggravate the srotas and the dhatus. Overeating, eating before the previous meal is digested, eating non-compatible foods, excessive or too little exercise, too much heat or cold, excessive worry, and concussion or shock can all aggravate the srotas.

The Srotas

SROTA	ITS ROOT	WHAT IT CARRIES
1. Prana vaha srotas	Respiratory tract	Oxygen, vital force
2. Udaka vaha srotas	Palate, pancreas	Water, fluids
3. Anna vaha srotas	Stomach	Food
4. Rasa vaha srotas	Heart	Chyle, lymph, plasma
5. Rakta vaha srotas	Liver, spleen	Blood
6. Mamsa vaha srotas	Tendons, ligaments, skin	Ingredients of muscle tissue

7. Meda vaha srotas	Kidneys	Ingredients of fat tissue
8. Asthi vaha srotas	Hip bone	Ingredients of bone tissue
9. Majja vaha srotas	Bones, joints	Ingredients of bone
10. Shukra vaha srotas	Testes, ovaries	Semen, ovum
11. Mootra vaha srotas	Kidneys, bladder	Urine
12. Varco vaha srotas	Colon, rectum	Feces
13. Sweda vaha srotas	Fat tissues	Sweat glands, skin

The Body's Wisdom

Understanding the beautiful way your body functions will help you understand why incorporating lifestyle changes will make the next part of your life free from problems. From the mahabhutas, to the doshas, dhatus, ojas, srotas, and malas—all are important in maintaining health. The three doshas, Vata, Pitta and Kapha, function through their respective subdoshas. They then move through the seven tissue levels (dhatus) either nourishing them, or if imbalanced, accumulating as disease.

The normal health of the body is maintained by the seven dhatus that are supplied by the channels (srotas). The malas are the waste products eliminated by the physiology. Health results when these systems function together in harmony. Disease is the disturbance of these systems due to improper diet for your doshic type or improper exercise and failure to keep your body cleansed and rejuvenated.

Ill health in any area of your life is also related to the intellect—that element which discriminates—becoming caught up in the diversity of creation and forgetting about the unity which underlies everything. The intellect's failure to recall the underlying unity while becoming engrossed in the sequential manifestations of diversity is called *pragya-aparadh,* the mistake of the intellect. And it is said in the ancient texts that this mistake leads to disease or unhappiness in the physiology in a variety of ways.

The mind, which entertains thoughts, some healthful and some not, plays a large part in your overall health. That is why Maharishi Vedic Medicine always recommends the Transcendental Meditation program as a first step to bring full balance and integration to the intellect and mind. And this also has a profound impact on the physiology.

Again, the Transcendental Meditation technique, the proper diet for *your* body makeup, the proper exercise for *you*, and Maharishi Vedic Medicine specific recommendations and rejuvenation and purification treatments are all important to constantly create and maintain a healthy life.

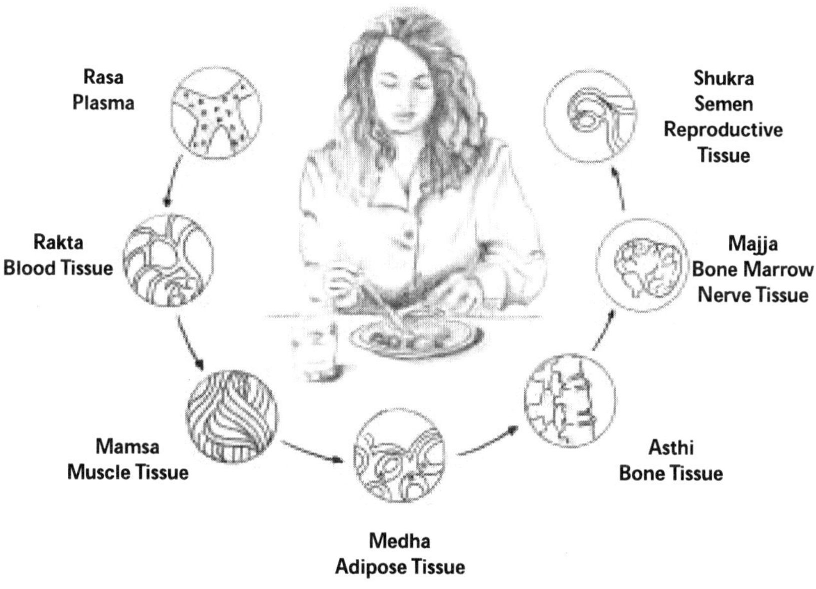

Circulation of nutrients and transformation of dhatus

References

1. Sharma, H. & Clark, C. 1998. *Contemporary Ayurveda*. Philadelphia: Churchill Livingstone, p. 46.
2. *Charaka Samhita*, Chikitsasthana 15:42-44.

Chapter Six

Understanding the Rhythms of Nature

Maharishi Vedic Medicine considers menopause to be a very special time of a woman's life—a time of wisdom, joy and attunement to one's inner Self. It is also the time for a woman to pay attention to keeping the body in a situation where toxins can be naturally released since she no longer has the advantage of the monthly purification of menstruation.

This is the time to incorporate a good daily routine, develop a good digestion, get regular exercise, and perform routines that help the circulation pick up the toxins in the physiology and remove them from the body. It is the time to tune in to the cycles of Mother Nature.

The Cycles of Mother Nature

Our bodies work best according to specific natural rhythms known as biological rhythms. Unfortunately, in our busy world we are heavily influenced by forces outside of our body that cause us to ignore our body's natural rhythms. For example, you may be tired and in need of sleep, yet your favorite television show is on; or you have a special event to attend, so you stay up, overriding your body's natural desire for sleep. This creates an imbalance in your body's natural rhythm. Or, you overeat—out of social influence, advertising influence, boredom or any number of influences that you allow to overrule your own natural inner intelligence and rhythm. At first the body is very forgiving and compensates. But, over time, the body gets tired of that strain and that strain shows up as an imbalance.

Keeping unnatural routines of staying up too late, overeating, or under exercising, can weaken the body's immune system. All too often busy women are doing all of them. If you have this unhealthy routine and you start menopause, your body is going to be very confused about what to do, unless you assist it by bringing your daily routine back into line with the rhythms of Mother Nature. Maharishi Vedic Medicine helps you attune your own biological rhythms to the rhythms of nature.

The Importance of Cycles

All biological rhythms or cycles are interrelated. Activity like travel, quiet activity like sleeping, even the activity of digestion—these can all affect your body's own natural rhythm.

If the body is trying to do one thing while you are trying to do something else, then imbalance occurs. You know through experience that an activity cycle doesn't mix well with a digestion cycle. "I couldn't sleep because I had too much for supper." "I can't go swimming because I just ate lunch."

In our own physiology of cycles, doshas have their own times of day. We know that these cycles will affect the patterns of our other biological cycles. If we align ourselves with the natural tendencies of these doshas, then things go smoothly.

The Concept of Daily Cycles

One way in which Maharishi Vedic Medicine promotes health is by bringing back a person's routine into synchrony with nature's rhythms.

There are many cultures around the world who recognize cycles in nature: annual, seasonal and monthly cycles. Some cycles are millennia long, some we would never notice in our lifetime, such as the 24,000-year cycle of the wobble of the earth.

The study of biological rhythms is known in modern medicine as chronobiology *(chronos* = time; *bios* = life; *logos* = science*)* or the rhythms of life. All life on earth, including our bodies, responds rhythmically to the regular cycles of the sun, moon, and seasons. These cycles influence almost every aspect of bodily functioning. For example, as the sun starts to rise, vital body functions, including heart rate and blood pressure, speed up in anticipation of increased physical activity. These and other predictable fluctuations in body function, taking place during specific time cycles, are our biological rhythms. They are regulated by "biological clock" mechanisms located in the brain.

Although biological rhythms can be disturbed by environmental influences, such as when a person regularly works the night shift and sleeps during the day, they are genetically programmed into our cells, tissues, and organs. One study showed that night shift workers have more medical disorders but they improved when they went back to day shifts.[1]

Modern medical chronobiologists have found that biologic rhythms can affect the severity of one's ills or the body's response to drug therapy. According to one study, a diseased tooth is most likely to begin aching between 3 and 8 a.m., and least likely to ache between 3 and 4 p.m.[2]

Formally known as the circadian rhythm, the 24-hour day/night–activity/rest cycle is also referred to as the "body clock." Many of our normal body functions follow daily patterns of speeding up and slowing down, intensifying and diminishing, in alignment with circadian rhythm. Many diseases are known by Western medicine to be more prominent at certain times of the day. Heart attacks and stroke most commonly occur in early waking hours while osteoarthritis symptoms flare up in the late afternoon and early evening.

Maharishi Vedic Medicine relates the biorhythms of the human body to an underlying regulator of biological rhythm. These not only influence the human body, but are throughout nature as well, and involve the three doshas of Vata, Pitta and Kapha.

Vata, Pitta and Kapha each regulate parts of the day of our daily cycles. Knowledge of the daily cycles is useful, and when you learn them, you can deal with them on a daily basis. You will find that when you are in tune with the daily cycles, it is like being in harmony with a great orchestra. Not following the daily cycles is like being out of tune.

Influences of Vata, Pitta and Kapha in Your 24-Hour Cycle

The three doshas break up the day for us like a clock—

Between 2 a.m to 6 a.m. and 2 p.m. to 6 p.m., Vata reigns.

Between 6 a.m. to 10 a.m. the qualities associated with Kapha dominate the environment and again from 6 p.m. to 10 p.m.

Between 10 a.m. to 2 p.m. and 10 p.m. to 2 a.m., Pitta reigns.

This concept is based on when the sun is rising, peaking and setting—the natural influence of the doshas. Since it's a concept, it doesn't matter if it's daylight savings time or not or where you live. It's general, so that you can make use of it without having to check the clock all the time.

2 to 6 a.m. or p.m. is Vata's cycle

Some of the old sayings are true: "Early to bed early to rise, makes a man *and a woman,* healthy, wealthy and wise." And, "The early bird gets the worm." In Maharishi Vedic Medicine the human being is part of nature, not outside of nature. The Vata time of the morning is one of stirring and awakening slightly before the sun comes up when all of nature is waking up.

Remember, Vata represents the following qualities: light, dry, airy, moving and consciousness. If you get up before 6 a.m., or before sunrise in Vata's cycle, the mind and body will reflect the best qualities of Vata—lightness, alertness and quickness. You will feel more alert and clear during the day. If you want lightness of body and lightness of personality, then you get up with the Vata dosha. If you sleep past sunrise and wake up in Kapha's cycle, then the body takes on the heaviness, slowness and dullness of Kapha. Wake up bright during Vata time and make good decisions all day long.

When Vata's cycle comes around at 2 p.m. to 6 p.m., and you haven't overeaten at lunch, which dulls the digestion and makes you tired, you will feel more energetic and ready for an active evening. Vata the mover takes things in and distributes them throughout the physiology. A very nice time to do your afternoon Transcendental Meditation is Vata time because of Vata's association with consciousness.

6 to 10 a.m. or p.m. is Kapha's cycle

Kapha is the heavy, slow, oily, dense, sturdy, immune, enduring, settled, regal dosha. If you awake during Kapha time, you will carry these slower, sleepier qualities throughout the day. The later you sleep the more sluggish you feel and the harder it is to get going. This makes it more likely to head for the coffee pot. It's as if you can't quite wake up and you need some outside stimulation.

Exercise during the Kapha time will stimulate Kapha. If you give stimulation to the body with exercise, the pounds will come off and stay off.

The 6 p.m. to 10 p.m. Kapha time is the ideal time to go to bed. If you get to bed during Kapha time (before 10 p.m.), it will be easier to fall asleep and sleep will be more restful, because it is dominated by Kapha's qualities of heaviness and tranquility. At this point, if you are listening to the body, then you will take this heavy, silent, nature of Kapha into sleep with you. Sleep will be quiet, deep, nourishing and satisfying. Western culture doesn't support this, because of electric lights, parties and television. You are going to have to make it your own priority.

10 to 2 a.m. or p.m. is Pitta's cycle

Pitta is in charge of digestion, metabolism, heat, and focused energy. From 10 a.m. to 2 p.m. the sun reaches its zenith and the day warms up. Eating lunch at Pitta's zenith (noon) is the perfect time to eat because the digestion and metabolism in the body is at its strongest. There is a correlation between the height of the sun and digestion. Digestion is more efficient when the sun is highest.

After 10 p.m. Pitta energy is rising again, this time for the purpose of internal purification and detoxification. If you are up and active after 10 p.m. you get your second wind. Then, instead of sleeping, you want to get up and do something. Instead of the body doing its nightly maintenance of house cleaning, toxins will build up over time. If you are up during the evening Pitta cycle, from 10 p.m. to 2 a.m., you will dissipate the body's own natural energy that it uses for internal cleansing into outward activity. You may notice when you stay up late that you also get hungry—this is because Pitta is rising. But Pitta is not rising to digest food, because at night this energy goes instead to the tissues for cleansing. If you eat during nighttime Pitta, you are creating ill health due to toxic build-up.

Begin the Day with Purification

Because the body is busy at night throwing off accumulated waste, your first morning activities should involve purification—the removal of the waste products that have accumulated in the previous evening.

Maharishi Vedic Medicine recommends beginning the day by evacuating the bowels, which eliminates the toxins and waste products of the previous day. Like getting up early or going to bed on time, this is a habit that over time you can train yourself to do.

Next, brush your teeth and gently scrape accumulated phlegm off the tongue with a special metal tongue scraper. Gargle with warm water and then sesame oil. This may sound strange until you understand how important gargling with sesame oil is to the health of your gums. Since aging brings on problems with teeth and especially gums, adding this simple technique into your daily routine should be a priority.

Why use sesame oil in particular? Dr. Edwards Smith first became interested in the use of sesame oil when he visited a Maharishi Ayur-Veda Health Center for treatment. He decided to study its effects on bacteria that grew in the mouth before and after a sesame oil mouth rinse. In a study undertaken on dental hygiene students at Wichita State University it was found that people who used a sesame oil gargle daily had significantly lower mouth bacteria.[3] Sesame oil helps prevent dental problems, especially periodontal or gum disease.

How to gargle with sesame oil:

- Rinse the mouth and throat with warm water. Gargle with warm water. Take a small mouthful of warm sesame oil (in other words, not so much that you gag). Hold the warm sesame oil in your mouth for one to two minutes. Then spit it out.
- Take a smaller amount of sesame oil, about half a mouthful. Gargle for one to two minutes, stopping for breath when necessary. Spit out. This helps protect the throat from soreness. It also loosens Kapha from the throat area. You may find that after you gargle with sesame oil, phlegm will come up into your throat which you can spit out.
- Next, using your finger, massage the gums in front of the teeth with sesame oil for a minute or two. Massage stimulates the gums and helps the sesame oil get absorbed.
- As the final step, rinse the mouth and throat with warm water again.

A Bit about Exercise

Although diet and exercise, with an emphasis on Maharishi Yoga asanas, will be covered more thoroughly in another chapter, it is mentioned here because you can incorporate moderate exercise into your morning routine. "Moderate" means you should exercise to one half of your capacity. The same goes for lifting weights (recommended for Kapha types). Morning is an ideal time for physical exercise because it is the Kapha period from sunrise to 10 a.m. when the body is feeling sluggish and needs the circulation to get going. The second best time is in the afternoon. The good advice to stay out of the sun between 10 a.m. and 2 p.m. can be applied to exercise, too. Pitta time, which tends to heat you anyway, is not a time to generate even more heat.

The evening is not considered a good time for strenuous exercise because it is too stimulating before sleep. Walking, however, especially after the evening meal, is considered by Maharishi Vedic Medicine to be health-promoting.

The next part of the morning routine is called *abhyanga*, a self-massage using warm sesame oil. This light oil massage is followed by a warm shower or bath. The sesame oil self-massage removes impurities from the tissues, then the shower or bath further removes them from the body.

The Benefits of Massage

Dr. Tiffany Field has researched the health benefits of massage.[4] The following is a brief list of the many benefits she has found from massage:

- Decreases the stress hormones cortisol and norepinephrine, thus calming the sympathetic nervous system.
- Increases vagal tone, the part of the parasympathetic nervous system that helps us rest and repair.
- Decreases substance P, a neurotransmitter that is increased when

one is in pain.

- Enhances the ability to perform at work.
- Increases the brain secretion of serotonin, thereby enhancing mood.

According to Maharishi Vedic Medicine, abhyanga has profound health benefits. The ancient Vedic texts on Ayur-Veda say that it promotes softness and luster of the skin, lubricates the muscles, tissues and joints, and increases their flexibility. By stimulating the tissues in the body, oil massage helps keep impurities from accumulating in the system. The texts also say that daily abhyanga make one less affected by old age.

How to Perform the Daily Oil Self-Massage

Because, after menopause, the body is no longer eliminating toxins through the blood as it did during menstruation and because our polluted environment puts an additional overload of toxins in our system, a daily warm oil self-massage should be added to your daily routine.

A daily self-massage can be done as quickly as rubbing perfumed lotion on your body and will produce many more benefits. It is not only an energizing way to start the day, it also helps you stay alert by stimulating all the organs of the body, getting a sluggish circulation flowing faster, and keeping the skin moist and subtle. Self-massage, and indeed, the massage used in Maharishi Ayur-Veda Health Centers throughout the world, has too many health benefits to ignore.

Cured warm sesame oil (unprocessed, cold-pressed, organic) is recommended for most body types. Generally, sesame oil is used in Maharishi Ayur-Veda massage because of its ability to reduce Vata's restlessness, increase Pitta's heat which is necessary for purification, and increase Kapha which calms the physiology, allowing it to relax. It also is a natural antiseptic and easily penetrates into the skin—more so than some other oils. When you are given an abhyanga at a Maharishi Ayur-Veda Health Center, specific herbs are recommended by the physician to help in specific treatments. Sesame oil has been found to carry these herbs most easily into the physiology because of its penetrating quality.

However, if you have a sensitivity to sesame seed or irritated skin with Pitta aggravations (redness, heat rash, breakouts), unprocessed, cold-pressed coconut oil can be substituted. Coconut oil decreases Vata and Pitta and increases Kapha.

Sweet almond oil is often recommended, especially in facial beauty treatments. Sweet almond oil increases Pitta, decreases Vata and Kapha.

Getting Ready for a Daily Oil Massage

Ideally, use cured, unprocessed, cold-pressed sesame oil for the massage. You can buy it in bulk at health food stores. The process of curing the oil only takes about five minutes and you can cure enough to last for several weeks.

To cure sesame oil, place up to one quart of it into a saucepan. Heat it to the boiling temperature of *water.* You don't need to boil the oil, which can be dangerous.

Use a candy thermometer to monitor the heat. As the oil begins to heat, the temperature will begin to rise more quickly. Watch the temperature very carefully. This is something you can't leave unattended.

Once the temperature reaches 212 degrees Fahrenheit, the oil is cured and you should immediately remove it from the heat. Let it cool and then store your oil in a glass container. Sesame oil is popular in Maharishi Vedic Medicine because it readily penetrates into the skin. It is best to store it in glass and transfer a little of it at a time into a squeeze plastic bottle for your daily massage.

When to Give Yourself a Daily Oil Massage

Give yourself a massage before you take your morning shower or bath. This is so easy—the instructions take longer to read than to actually do it. Once you perform a couple of self-massages and have the instructions memorized, you'll find it easy to make it a part of your morning routine. You'll wonder how you ever lived without it.

Self-Massage Equals Self-Healing

Warm the oil slightly before the massage. This helps the oil sink in faster and also feels better to the skin. An easy way to warm the oil is to put it in a small plastic bottle and run hot water over it.

Apply a light covering of oil to each part of the body before massaging it—head, ears and face first.

Use an open palm rather than your fingertips. Use light pressure or pressure that feels good to you.

Using a circular motion, massage the top, side and back of your head with both hands. Gently massage the outer ears.

Circle the temples and cheeks. Stroke across the forehead, then the upper lip and chin.

Next massage the front and back of the neck, using horizontal strokes back and forth. Be extra gentle over the windpipe.

Massage each arm separately. Circle the shoulder, use long strokes back and forth on the upper arm; circle the elbow, and use long strokes back and forth on the lower arm. The method here is to use long strokes on the long bones and circular strokes on the joints.

Circle the wrist. Massage the palm of the hand and the back of the hand, then pull each finger gently.

Make circles on the breasts with both hands, using very gentle, circular motion over the heart.

Use a clockwise motion over the abdomen.

Next, use long strokes to massage up and down the spine and back, as far as you can reach.

Massage each leg separately, using long strokes on the upper leg, circular strokes on the knee and long strokes on the calf. Circle the ankles.

Finally the feet. Massage back and forth on the Achilles tendon, heel, and top of the foot. Use the palm of the hand to stroke lengthwise on the sole of the foot. Gently pull the toes.

Next, take your morning shower or bath. Bathing in warm water helps open the channels of circulation and allows the impurities that you have just loosened through the massage to flow into the digestive tract.

This daily massage is highly recommended and should be made a mandatory daily activity just as brushing your teeth. The health benefits far outweigh any reasons for skipping it.

The end of the morning purification routine is to practice the Transcendental Meditation technique and then eat a light breakfast.

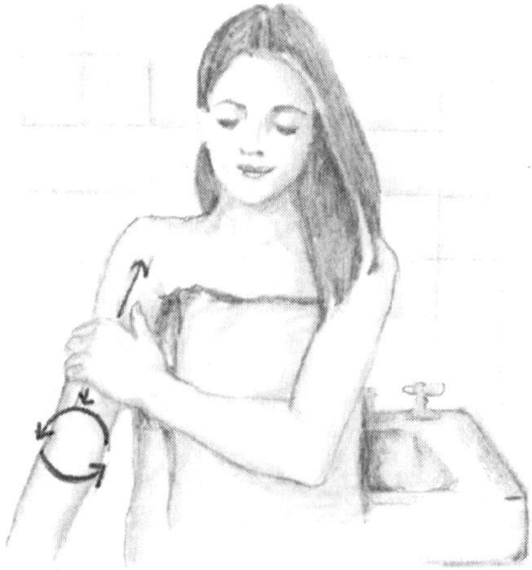

Performing abhyanga oil massage is an essential part of the daily routine. It strengthens and balances the whole physiology, improves circulation and vitality, and rejuvenates the skin.

Seasonal Influences

Each of the doshas has a corresponding season in which its influences are strongly felt in the physiology no matter which mind-body constitution you have. However, if it is Pitta season and you have accumulated Pitta in your physiology, then Pitta would be more easily aggravated.

Just a reminder here that it is important not to be confused by all the different influences of daily cycles, seasonal cycles or lifetime cycles. A Maharishi Vedic Medicine physician will check your imbalances and give you suggestions of what to do according to your mind-body constitution and with regard to seasonal changes. This will let you focus on your specific needs.

The seasonal changes in your environment during a year's time affect the three doshas. For this reason, your routine may adjust to incorporate the seasonal influences of Vata, Pitta and Kapha.

Vata is aggravated by the cold winds of late autumn and winter because Vata tends to be cold and dry. Pitta dosha, because it is hot and moist, is aggravated by summer's heat. Pitta season is midsummer to early autumn. The dosha that is aggravated by springtime's moisture and coolness is Kapha, because its qualities are already wet and cold. Kapha season, a wet and cooler time of year, is spring to early summer.

Maharishi Vedic Medicine knows that nature and the body are part of a single continuum of intelligence—the human body and the body of nature recognize each other. Since each season exhibits the predominance of one dosha, balancing the doshas is the key to adapting to their effects.

Winter's cold weather increases both Vata and Kapha because they are both cold. Vata, the most irregular and unpredictable dosha, needs special attention in its own season. Because Vata is quick-moving, it becomes aggravated immediately. Therefore, winter is an especially important time to follow a Vata-reducing diet and routine. Slow-moving Kapha increases more slowly, so spring is the ideal time to follow a Kapha-reducing diet. The hot summer is the time for a Pitta-reducing routine.

When the seasons change you will notice a shifting of the qualities of the doshas. For example, summer to autumn is Pitta season shifting to Vata season. Change aggravates Vata and Vata is the leader of the other two doshas. This change can be destabilizing to the physiology.

The influence of the destabilizing nature of seasonal changes is very noticeable from a medical perspective. Medical professionals often see that when the seasons change, people generally feel poorly. They can catch colds or the flu, have strep throat or similar health problems.

The routine recommended for a new season should be eased into gradually over a period of one or two weeks, just before the new season starts, so as not to aggravate Vata.

Vata Season—Late Autumn to Early Winter

Because menopause happens in the Vata time of life, it is especially important to incorporate Vata-pacifying factors into your daily routine. Vata season is late autumn to early winter. However, in Maharishi Vedic Medicine, autumn is not considered so much one season as the junction of two—Pitta season and Vata season. Pitta accumulates over the summer, therefore Pitta needs attention until middle or late October.

When cooler weather comes along a change occurs and Vata begins to dominate in the environment. Because any transition can aggravate Vata, and this particular transition is from Pitta (summer) to Vata's own season of autumn, it is doubly important to keep Vata balanced. The enlivenment of Vata can have good effects, especially if you tend to have a good deal of Kapha in your physiology, because Vata increases energy, vitality and liveliness. Some people feel that autumn is the best time of the year for them because they feel more "alive" at this time.

Vata types, however, can have a particularly hard time if Vata dosha becomes aggravated. They can become overly sensitive to cold, come down with respiratory infections, insomnia, dry skin, hyperactivity, indecisiveness and worry. These Vata factors are especially associated with aging.

To compensate for an excess of Vata in the physiology,

Maharishi Vedic Medicine favors warmth and oleation, the opposite of Vata's cold and dry qualities. It may seem obvious, but sometimes busy people can forget the obvious. By the way, the word "favors" means "to go towards." It does not mean you absolutely must incorporate everything you learn here at this moment. Use your common sense and adapt to the situation that you are in. If you are at a meal and are served foods that you feel are not suitable to your physiology, but you would insult the host or hostess if you didn't eat it—then eat it (at least some of it). Adapting to a situation shows flexibility.

Favoring warmth means:

- Eat warm, well-cooked foods. Eat warm, oilier foods. Favor foods with sweet, sour and salty tastes. Minimize cold, dry, raw, rough, pungent or astringent foods. This is not the time to get into a raw foods diet, because that will aggravate Vata.
- Stop drinking cold drinks; drink warm liquids instead.
- Keep well wrapped up, because the warmth of the body radiates through the skin. Keep the head and neck covered on windy, rainy or cold days and avoid drafts. Drafts especially aggravate Vata.
- Central heating can further dry the air indoors, so a humidifier is recommended.
- A daily warm oil self-massage is highly recommended.

Pitta Season—Midsummer through Early Autumn

In summer, exercise *less,* not more (as a lot of people do), because exercise heats the body which needs to stay cool in summer. Walking in the early morning and evening, swimming, and moderate exercise will help keep excess Pitta from building up. Premature aging of the skin and skin cancer can show up on those with excess Pitta and aggravated Pitta.

Since the eyes are one of the main seats of Pitta dosha

(Alochaka Pitta), the summer sun can aggravate them. Wearing sunglasses on bright summer days is recommended along with wearing a hat or using a parasol.

Sunbathing, however, is not recommended. According to Maharishi Vedic Medicine, ten minutes per day of direct exposure to the sun is enough.

What to Favor:

- Favor cool, astringent, sweet, bitter and oily foods; minimize hot, spicy, salty foods.
- Decrease the amount of exercise and don't stay out in the sun.
- Swim. Walk in cool places such as forests, mountains, gardens or in the evening moonlight.
- Wear a hat and sunglasses outdoors.

Kapha Season—Spring through Early Summer

During the colder winter weather Kapha accumulates in the physiology. When the weather warms up, Pitta "liquefies" the Kapha which is then eliminated from the body, usually in the form of mucus. This is known among Ayurvedic practitioners as a "Kapha meltdown."

Having a runny nose at the first signs of spring, nasal allergies, colds, coughs, sinusitis, and other respiratory congestion problems are all signs of Kapha aggravation. Its environmental equivalent is a frozen glacier melting.

A Kapha-pacifying diet of eating more foods with bitter, spicy, or astringent tastes and less foods that are sweet, cold, oil, heavy and salty will greatly pacify Kapha. (See the chapter on diet.)

During spring it is advised to drink warm liquids only and stay away from cold drinks. Sunshine helps reduce Kapha as does exercise. Exercise for Kapha types in the spring is especially important. Spring cleaning of the physiology is highly recommended at this time. Maharishi Ayur-Veda Health Centers have several programs of purification and rejuvenation (See the Index). If you have just entered into menopause, or are perimenopausal, taking purification and rejuvenation treatments at this time will definitely help keep you in healthy running order.

What to Favor:

- Exercise
- Favor warm food and drinks. Favor foods with spicy, astringent, and bitter tastes.
- Favor more activity and minimize daytime napping, which increases Kapha.

The Benefits of a Daily Routine

According to Maharishi Vedic Medicine you don't just wake up one day with a problem—you have developed it over time by straining the body slightly day after day. The body tries to compensate but eventually it says "I can't do this any more," and a symptom develops.

You strain the body by having an erratic schedule. Therefore, culture your physiology by giving it a healthy daily routine. Pick a time to eat, a time to get up and a time to go to sleep which are all in tune with nature.

During the early morning Vata cycle, 2 a.m. to 6 a.m, Vata the mover picks up waste products and moves them to various exit areas of the body. When you wake up during Vata time, you can eliminate these waste products through hygienic procedures that you have been taught to do since childhood.

If Vata the mover is allowed to do her job properly, then the first thing in the morning you should be able to empty your bladder and evacuate your bowels, naturally without strain. Other areas of the body eliminate their waste and also need attention in the morning. The mouth is an exit area and needs rinsing and the teeth, brushing; ears need cleaning; maybe the nose needs blowing if there is an excess of Kapha.

If you are not in the habit of getting up before 6 a.m., you can easily culture the body to wake up at that time even without an alarm. Here is a little experiment you can do to support your desire for better health. Set your alarm for 5:55 a.m. The first couple of days you will be annoyed that you had to be disturbed by the alarm. But by the third day or so you will wake up a few minutes before the alarm goes off because the mind doesn't like it. (Be sure to get to bed early enough the night before.)

It's the same principle as in the case of evacuating the bowels. After a while the body will be trained to have a bowel evacuation. The body loves to be cultured like that, when it is being gently guided into a more healthful routine. Balancing the Vata dosha is simply a matter of creating a routine.

These early morning cleansing routines are not to be ignored in the name of "being natural." It is healthy and wise to cleanse the skin, mouth, teeth and areas where bacteria can build up.

Maharishi Vedic Medicine considers menstruation to be a way that a woman's body is naturally cleansed once a month. When it stops, it is then even more important for her to help her body stay healthy with a good daily routine and internal cleansing programs taken at Maharishi Ayur-Veda Health Centers.

Those with predominant Pitta dosha should ideally incorporate everything they learn into their daily routines immediately. This is a worthy goal but can be somewhat overwhelming. Instead, pick a couple of things during the day that allow you to start a good routine. Change gradually. The body likes to be coaxed gently.

One of the most important things is to eat your largest meal at noon when Pitta is at its peak. Again, you can culture the body to do this. To get the most efficient digestion you can aim to eat by 12:30. Do this and the body will start getting the digestive enzymes ready around 12:15. If you are not culturing the body (and the mind) to eat at a specific time, and you put food in the body, it will not have the digestive enzymes ready. The result is inefficient digestion.

Also, the opposite is true. If you ignore the needs of the body when it is hungry, after a while the body will digest something else—the stomach lining maybe. It's very important to listen to the language of the body.

An Ayurvedic good day starts the night before during Kapha time when you naturally start to tire. But if you have been staying up past Kapha time into Pitta time, then you have to gradually retrain your body to go to bed earlier. Don't strain. The body doesn't like to be changed quickly, so change at a comfortable rate. Gradually change from going to bed at midnight (if that's been your habit) to going to bed at 11:45 p.m. Then 11:30, and so forth, until you get to 9 or 9:30 p.m.

Know that there is a dynamic influence or relationship between Vata, Pitta and Kapha doshas. They work together and must all be kept in balance. Pitta cuts the denseness of Kapha because Pitta is heat. An everyday example is found in the use of detergent which has a bit of lemon in it. Lemon is an astringent and has Pitta qualities—it cuts the dense dirt-like qualities that are Kapha. If you eat hot and spicy foods, your nose starts to run. This is an example of the "hot spice" of Pitta melting Kapha.

Another way to remember the dynamic relationship between the three doshas is to think of your digestion as a campfire. In order to have a campfire you have to have fire (Pitta), a log (Kapha) and oxygen (Vata). It is the proper balance between the three that keeps the campfire burning brightly. First, oxygen is needed or the fire won't burn. If there is too little, the fire goes out, or if there is too much, the fire goes out. The same thing happens with reference to the amount of wood or fuel used to maintain the fire—too large a log will snuff out the fire; but by the same token, if there is not enough fuel, the fire has nothing to burn and will go out. Vata, Pitta and Kapha must stay in balance in order to have a good "fire of digestion."

These Changes Will Change Your Life

Although most of these suggestions may seem obvious, it is surprising how many people forget the "basics" or are too busy to attend to themselves. At this time of your life, you need to synchronize yourself with the rhythms of nature. Instead of swimming up river against the current, it is time to learn to surf the waves. The result? You'll feel that life is a joy.

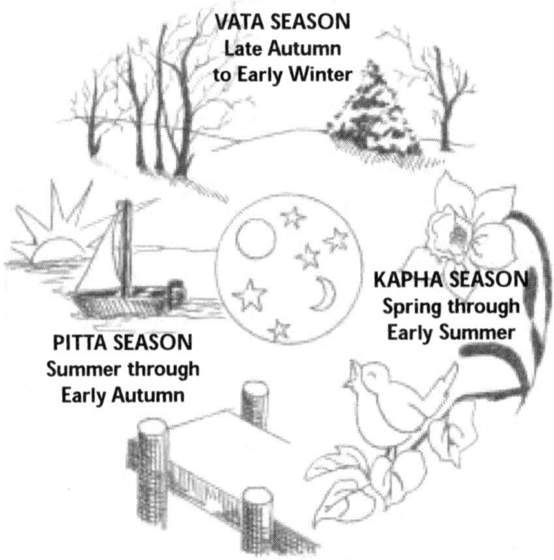
VATA SEASON
Late Autumn
to Early Winter
KAPHA SEASON
Spring through
Early Summer
PITTA SEASON
Summer through
Early Autumn

The seasons classfied according to the doshas

References

1. Meers, A., Maasen, A. & Verhaegen, P. 1978. Subjective health after six months and after four years of shift work. *Ergonomics,* 21, 857–859.
2. Pollmann, L. & Harris, P.H.P. 1978. Rhythmic changes in pain sensitivity in teeth. *International 1 Journal of Chronobiology,* 5, 459–464.
3. Stevens, M.M. 1989 (June). *The effects of a sesame oil mouth rinse on the number of oral bacteria colony types.* Presented at the 11th

International Symposium on Dental Hygiene, Ottawa, Canada.

4. Field, T. et al. 1997. Massage therapy effects on depression and somatic symptoms in chronic fatigue syndrome, *Journal of Chronic Fatigue Syndrome*, 3, 43–51.

Chapter Seven

Food Is the Best Medicine

The *Surgeon General's Report on Nutrition and Health* states, "For the two out of three adult Americans who do not smoke and do not drink excessively, one personal choice seems to influence long-term health prospects more than any other: what we eat."[1]

Your body constitution along with your special dietary needs determine your eating habits. Your eating habits are very important in determining what the rest of your life will be like, health-wise.

At the onset of menopause women need to understand how they can prevent rapid aging. Even though menopause may not seem connected to diet, it is. Every aspect of the physiology is connected to every other aspect of the physiology. If one part is not functioning properly, then every other part is affected.

According to the ancient Ayur-Veda texts, the distinction between health and disease arises as the result of the difference between a wholesome and unwholesome diet. In other words, disease is the result of faulty nutrition. The value of getting proper nutrients can't be over emphasized along with the fact that you need to digest them properly. If you eat healthy, organic foods and are able to digest them properly then your body will have a natural access to a whole pharmacy of healthy nutrients. As Jean Carper points out in *The Food Pharmacy*, "We are talking about a food pharmacy of unimaginable versatility and complexity, made up of natural laxatives, tranquilizers, beta blockers, antibiotics, anticoagulants, antidepressants, painkillers, cholesterol reducers, anti-inflammatory agents, hypotensives, analgesics, decongestants, digestives, expectorants, anti-motion sickness agents, cancer inhibitors, antioxidants, contraceptives, vasodilataos and vasoconstrictors, anticavity agents, antiulcerataive agents, insulin regulators, to name a few."[2]

Diet and Digestion

How does digestion relate to menopause? Vata, Pitta and Kapha doshas are all governed by the quality of the foods you take into your physiology. Too many hot foods and Pitta dosha becomes aggravated—that can set off hot flashes. If Kapha is out of balance due to dietary influences, cysts and tumors can develop. The thin Vata-type woman is susceptible to osteoporosis.

One of the primary concerns of Maharishi Vedic Medicine is the ability to digest food properly. In Maharishi Vedic Medicine the knowledge of diet is organized around four major principles:

- Proper nutrition (diet) can be used as therapeutic remedies
- Taste is a guide to food's nutritional value
- Your principle dosha determines which foods are best for you
- How you eat is as important as what you eat

Food as Therapy

Maharishi Vedic Medicine understands that the body is more than just physical matter. It is, in fact, a dynamic network of energy and intelligence. Food, also, is a network of energy and intelligence. The proper diet, chosen according to your mind-body type, will keep the body's network in balance. As mentioned before, maintaining the body's balance is considered by Maharishi Vedic Medicine as the basis of health. The primary tool you can use for maintaining health is your diet even if no nutritional deficiencies show up in Western medical tests.

Many women use food as an emotional weapon, a means to

insulate themselves with fat or get attention by becoming too thin. They even use food to slowly commit suicide by constantly eating improperly. If you've been sabotaging your health by using food incorrectly, it is time now—now or never—to switch your thinking. If you want to feel badly for the rest of your life—ignore your diet. On the other hand, develop an understanding of how eating the food that is best for your mind-body type will promote health and help eliminate problems associated with menopause. As you follow the recommendations of Maharishi Vedic Medicine, you'll find that your mind and body are more in tune with nature, and you'll naturally enjoy the foods that are good for you.

The Importance of Taste

The human body is an intricate ecosystem—food affects the balance of every area of the body. Many factors can influence your diet: the time of day something is eaten, the state of balance or imbalance of your body, what time of the year it is, and what your mental conditioning is towards certain foods. Even our daily experiences become part of our "diet."

According to Maharishi Vedic Medicine we take in or "metabolize" our experiences and our ideas, which then become metabolized into our cellular structure. Everything you do and experience—at home, work, and play—can alter the current state of balance in your physiology. As that state of balance changes, so should your diet. How can you know what you should eat at any given point of time? It's easy really. Pay attention to the sense of taste.

You might have read that in order to have a balanced diet you must get such-and-such amount of this or that vitamin a day. Or, you have to eat so much from a food pyramid—stuffing so much fruit, bread, meat and vegetables into your body. This will sometimes work (combined with an exercise program) to help you lose weight, because it helps you cut back on unnecessary fats and sugar. This is great but may not, ultimately, keep you healthy.

Western medicine has determined the "recommended daily allowances" of vitamins and minerals strictly from laboratory tests or observation of those who are sick—in other words, those who are in abnormal states of health. Laboratory animals are deprived of certain nutrients until they develop a disease, or hospitals keep records of those people who already have deficiencies. Even prisoners volunteer to have nutritional tests performed on them. The data gathered from this type of testing can be valuable, but doesn't give the whole picture of what health and an ideal diet for each individual actually would be.

Historically, we humans, along with all creatures great and small, have used taste and smell to avoid toxic or unhealthy foods and to find nutritious ones.

Pregnant women's food cravings, based on taste and smell, are coming to be understood as a mechanism to protect the embryo.[3]

If food cravings have their basis in physiological need, then that craving is naturally balancing. When a pregnant woman or a child has indigestion or a deficiency, they don't ask for enzymes or vitamins, proteins or minerals, but crave something spicy, sour or sweet, etc., which shows that the body naturally has its own self-referral mechanism—it restores balance through cravings and desires. Saying spicy, sour or sweet does not mean junk food. Maharishi Vedic Medicine recognizes these different qualities in natural, wholesome foods.

The Six Taste Groups

All foods are classified by Maharishi Vedic Medicine as belonging to one or more of six taste groups. In order to have balance in your diet, you should have all six tastes at every meal. The six tastes are:

Sweet • Sour • Salty • Pungent • Bitter • Astringent

Unfortunately, a Western diet favors only the three tastes of sweet, sour and salty. These three tastes increase Kapha dosha which leads to obesity.

Sweet

Of course, sugary foods are sweet, but usually the Western diet has too many of these "sweets"—and they have all sorts of other fattening goodies included. For example, let's look at a product marketed as a snack cake. Aside from sugar, the product includes corn syrup, vegetable shortening, flour, cocoa, eggs, soybean oils, salt, emulsifiers, artificial colors and artificial flavors. Simply not a good way to satisfy your taste for sweets.

In Maharishi Vedic Medicine "sweet" includes: milk, grains, bread, cooked starchy tubers (potatoes and sweet potatoes), some vegetables, and sweet fruits.

Sour

If you think of the word "sour," your mouth usually puckers up at the thought of lemons, or other sour citrus fruits. But also included in the sour taste group are: yogurt, cheese, other curdled milk products, fermented substances, carbonated beverages and tomatoes.

Salty

What constitutes a salty taste is obvious: any kind of salt and food to which large amounts of salt have been added—salty snack foods, pickles, sauerkraut.

Pungent

Cayenne, chili peppers, onions, garlic, radishes, ginger, spicy foods.

Bitter

Eggplant, turmeric, zucchini and leafy green vegetables.

Astringent

Astringent foods include those that have a drying quality, such as beans, pomegranates and apples, spinach, and green leafy vegetables.

To keep the doshas balanced, include something from each taste group in every meal, even if it's just a tiny amount—just a taste.

Why should you have all six tastes at every meal? Because the six tastes stimulate the proper sequence of the digestive process, and they add interest and diversity to meals. A deeper understanding shows that each taste has an effect on each dosha, to either increase it or decrease it. Therefore, taste acts as a balancing mechanism for your physiology.

If you understand how the doshas work, you will be able to eat according to which dosha needs increasing or decreasing. For example, as you already know, sweet, sour and salty increases Kapha. If you are trying to gain weight, choose sweet, sour and salty foods. They increase Kapha. Then what do they decrease? Vata. That makes sense, because Kapha has the quality of heaviness and Vata the quality of lightness. To have the opposite effect (decrease Kapha and increase Vata) pungent, bitter and astringent tastes are chosen. A pungent food like ginger increases the appetite; a bitter food like green, leafy vegetables is light in calories, high in vitamins; and an astringent food, such as honey, will add sweetness without empty calories. All of these foods make sense if you are trying to lose weight, because they decrease Kapha and increase lightness.

Sweet, bitter and astringent tastes decrease Pitta while the sour, salty and pungent tastes increase Pitta. If you know someone who is in a fiery Pitta rage, what food would you hand them? Something sweet and cool like ice cream. Calms them right down. Hot flashes are an obvious imbalance of Pitta. Cutting down on the sour, salty and pungent foods along with taking balancing Maharishi Ayur-Veda herbs helps with hot flashes.

Conversely, if you want to put a little fire under someone to get him or her moving, you'll want to increase Pitta and decrease Kapha with something pungent, like spicy food. Just remember, everyone needs some of all six tastes but not necessarily in equal amounts. Those who want to decrcase Vata should eat more sweet and fewer astringent foods, but should still have some of both.

How the Tastes Affect the Doshas

Sweet, sour, salty—increases Kapha, decreases Vata
Pungent, bitter, astringent—decreases Kapha, increases Vata
Pungent, sour, salty—increases Pitta
Sweet, bitter, astringent—decreases Pitta

Maharishi Vedic Medicine does not rely solely on taste to balance the physiology, but it does regard taste as a major guide for balancing an individual's diet. The balance of one's ideal tastes depends on her body type.

Your Principle Dosha Determines Foods That Are Best for You

In Maharishi Vedic Medicine the principle of "like increases like, and opposites decrease opposites" is used in dietary advice for pacifying Vata, Pitta and Kapha doshas.

Vata dosha is dry and cold; therefore, the opposite qualities of oily and warm foods will have a calming effect.

Specifically, a Vata-pacifying diet would be:

Favor foods that are:	*Reduce* foods that are:
warm	cold
oily	dry
heavy	light
sweet	spicy
sour	bitter
salty	astringent

Pitta dosha is hot and acidic, therefore, to pacify Pitta eat more cold and sweet foods.

Specifically, a Pitta-pacifying diet would be:

Favor foods that are:	*Reduce* foods that are:
cold	warm
heavy	light
oily	dry
sweet	spicy
bitter	salty
astringent	sour

Kapha is cold and oily, therefore, spicy, pungent foods are recommended.

Specifically, a Kapha-pacifying diet would be:

Favor foods that are:	*Reduce* foods that are:
light	heavy
dry	oily
warm	cold
spicy	sweet
bitter	salty
astringent	sour

Of course, since everyone is a combination of doshas—Vata/Pitta, Kapha/Pitta, Vata/Kapha, etc.—a mixed diet is advised. For example, a Vata/Pitta should pay attention to both doshas' diets, with more Vata-pacifying foods eaten in the windy winter and with more emphasis on the Pitta diet in the Pitta-aggravating heat of summer.

Notice that the recommendations say "favor" and "reduce," not "only eat" and "never eat." If you have "only" and "never" in your diet, then you will become out of balance. Balance is the key to good health. Several Ayurvedic cookbooks are out on the market, which will help clarify what to eat.

When to Eat, How Much to Eat and How to Eat

When

Eating your main meal at noon during Pitta time will use your maximum digestive fire. "Digestive fire" is the digestive system's overall ability to digest—when the enzymes are ready to go to work. The term digestive fire in Maharishi Vedic Medicine is known as "agni." (We discussed the thirteen agnis as principles of transformation from one dhatu to another.) If your agni is strong, then you will have few digestive problems. If it is weak, then you won't digest your food properly. Pitta types usually have strong agni. Vata types' agni varies. And Kapha types have slow or dull agni. As long as agni is functioning properly, the process of breaking down food and absorbing and assimilating it into the body will operate smoothly.

Don't eat again until the meal is fully digested—usually two and a half hours later or longer. Otherwise, you'll have some food that is "cooked" by the digestive enzymes and some that is not. This creates *ama*—a toxic residue that will be explained in a moment. You can tell when the meal is fully digested, because you will become hungry. If you aren't hungry, don't eat.

Keep regular meal times—a regular routine helps the body digest better. (See tips in the chapter on daily routine.)

How Much to Eat

The agni or digestive enzymes need some room in the kitchen of your digestive tract to work. Therefore, don't fill it completely full. Eat slowly and pay attention to your eating, so that when you feel satisfied—not stuffed or full, but satisfied—stop eating. This allows digestion to be complete. You're an adult, so you don't have to go by that old childhood rule of "clean your plate." When you are satisfied, put down your eating utensil and push your plate away.

A general rule of thumb: eat an amount that is equivalent to the amount that two cupped hands can hold. Don't load your plate as if this were the last meal that you are ever going to eat. Or, don't put such a tiny amount on your plate that you feel deprived just looking at it.

How to Eat

According to Maharishi Vedic Medicine it is better to eat in a settled atmosphere. This means no fast-food meals while driving, no lunch at your desk while discussing business, no watching TV. Set a nice table, sit down, say a blessing or grace if it is your custom, and eat quietly.

Why do people eat incorrectly? What is at the basis of hunger or desire for one or the other food? The emotions have a very powerful effect on the physiology. If you are being ruled by your emotions, you should wait a while before eating. Upsetting emotions greatly influence the physiology, so don't ingest them. Don't eat when angry, upset or disturbed emotionally in any way.

- Sit down to eat—no eating out of the refrigerator or eating over the sink, walking around with your cell phone, etc. Sit!
- Don't talk while chewing food. Get off that phone while eating! Not only does it interfere with digestion, it is very rude to chew in someone's ear. Nice, quiet conversations with family and friends is okay. Understand that chewing well and swallowing before speaking helps predigest the food.
- Avoid taking milk with meals that have mixed tastes. You can drink milk at other times. In Maharishi Vedic Medicine, cow's milk, drunk separately and properly heated, is considered a healthy food. This, too, will be discussed in a later chapter.
- Favor fresh, wholesome foods. This means organic, whenever possible, even if, or especially if, you are a vegetarian. If you aren't eating organic, you are putting pesticides and herbicides into your body.
- Favor cooked foods over raw foods. This can be a switch for you if you've lived your life eating lots of raw salads. Raw foods advocates feel that cooking food results in a loss of nutrients. In Maharishi Vedic Medicine, it is important to ingest adequate nutrients. But here is the reasoning for eating cooked food:

cooked foods are easier to digest, because cooking is the first step in the process of digestion. Minor nutrient losses in cooking will be more than compensated for, because the body will find the remaining nutrients easier to assimilate. Naturally ripened fruit, which has been cooked by the sun, is considered cooked food. Unfortunately, many fruits found in grocery stores are not sun-ripened.

- Avoid cold drinks. Cold drinks douse the digestive fire. Sip moderate amounts of warm, or room temperature, water with meals. In hot weather, cool drinks are okay, especially for those with Pitta constitutions.
- After eating, stay seated for four or five minutes. This allows the digestion to begin. Western medicine agrees that there is a blood shunt to the digestive tract during this time. You have a choice between jumping up from the table or properly digesting your food—it's healthier at this time to sit quietly and allow digestion to take place.

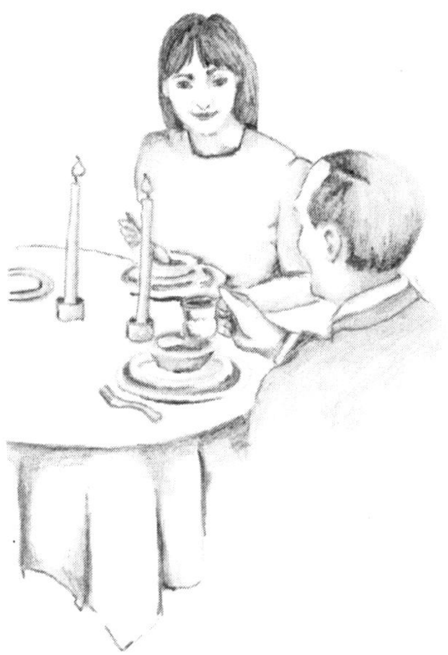

Eating in a settled atmosphere helps aid digestion.

All about Ama

Ama is a sticky toxic material that collects in the body and is the end-product of poorly digested food. It is as if your undigested food has turned into sticky glue. This putrefied food clogs the channels in the body, which starts you on the way to disease.

You can actually see if ama is accumulating in your body. First thing in the morning stick out your tongue while looking in the mirror. If there is a white, greenish or brown coating on the tongue which can be scraped off, that coating is ama. This sticky substance can clog your digestive system where most disease starts. Because ama contributes to the early stage of many diseases, Maharishi Vedic Medicine considers reducing ama of the utmost importance. Once ama is formed how do you get rid of it? By promoting good digestion you lessen the production of ama.

Not only is ama considered to be a toxin, but unnatural chemicals in food, air, water, building materials and some medicines are toxic as well. Besides having a coating of ama on the tongue, other signs of toxic accumulation are:

bad breath
skin problems—pimples, rashes, age spots
congestion and excess mucus
allergies
odors from stools and urine
unpleasant body odors

Toxins in the body can inhibit or impair normal metabolic functioning. Maharishi Vedic Medicine considers toxic build-up the root cause of most chronic disease.

Helping Prevent Ama Build-Up

- Eat during Pitta time when the digestive fire is high. It is highest at noon. Low digestive fire is considered to be behind the accumulation of toxins in the body and most digestive disorders.

- Eat fresh ginger one half hour before a meal (if you aren't excessively Pitta prone).
- Pay attention to all six tastes. Using all six tastes at lunch and dinner promotes better digestion.
- Drink plain hot water if you are not excessively Pitta. Drinking hot water mobilizes ama. But if you have too much Pitta or the weather is too hot, drink warm water or room temperature water.
- Use a tongue scraper on the front part of the tongue where the fine bumps are, not too far back where the large bumps are, to scrape off ama.
- Perform a daily oil self-massage that helps loosen toxins and ama from the system. (See the section on daily routine.)
- Eat fresh, wholesome food.
- For relief of uncomfortable menopause symptoms, take fresh, organic aloe vera gel, one teaspoon three times a day.
- If toxins are not being eliminated properly, check with your physician who is trained in Maharishi Ayur-Veda to get some helpful pointers and/or a recommendation of Maharishi Ayur-Veda herbs that will mobilize ama.
- Perform Maharishi Ayur-Veda purification and rejuvenation treatments.

The Benefits of Drinking Pure Warm Water

In most articles on diet these days, the writer mentions drinking eight to ten glasses of water a day. What they fail to mention is that it should be hot, or at least warm, pure water, and not cold, or ice, water.

Why warm water? You drink warm water because warm water most efficiently washes out your internal pipes and aids in digestion. You don't wash dishes in cold water, because it is hot water that helps easily remove food from the dishes. Same principle at work.

Hot water not only keeps the gastrointestinal tract flushed, but it keeps your body well-hydrated. Cold water or ice water will constrict the digestive tract and even put out the digestive fire—because it's cold and cold constricts. Heat relaxes.

Although drinking herbalized teas and other healthy drinks are good, too, drinking enough pure water is what keeps the body flushed. Teas, fruit drinks, or anything else but pure water, will be metabolized by the body as a food. If you retain water (imbalanced Kapha physiologies have a tendency toward this), this is a good indication that your body needs plain water to flush out toxins.

Take the time to buy either natural spring water, or to get a purifier for your home water supply. These days even small convenience stores carry bottled water. If you buy it, let it warm up. Look around you at airports or activity centers. You will see many health-conscious people carrying bottled water or thermoses of water.

Create Ojas in Your Physiology

Ojas is a biochemical substance that permeates your entire physiology. As mentioned before, ojas is the end-product of perfect digestion and metabolism, but there is even more to it. It also is considered by Ayurvedic texts to connect consciousness and matter and to nourish and sustain the various dhatus.[5] When the amount of ojas becomes too low, then life itself is threatened.

When there is an abundance of ojas in your physiology, it gives physical strength, immune strength, contentment, and good digestion. Ojas also appears on the skin as a radiant glow. The texts consider ojas to be the most important biochemical substance mediating the influence of consciousness on the body.

There are two types of ojas, ordinary and superior. The texts say that superior ojas exists in eight drops in *hridaya* (heart). Hridaya deals with the link between the emotions and their effects on the physiology, which is discussed in the chapter on emotions.

It is important at this stage in your life to make sure you have plenty of ojas. Maharishi Vedic Medicine lists the following methods to increase ojas:

- The main factor determining ojas production is the level of your consciousness. This means that the more you are "awake" and happy as a result of practicing Transcendental Meditation and following a good routine, the more ojas is spontaneously produced.

- Good digestion and a balanced diet of pure, wholesome foods helps improve the production of ojas. Some foods increase ojas and others decrease it. That does not mean that you should eat only these foods. A balanced diet is always recommended that includes *some* of these foods. Some ojas producing foods are:
    - milk
    - ghee (clarified butter)
    - rice (organic)
    - sweet fruits
    - dates and raisins

The ancient writings of Ayurveda also examine qualities of ojas and alcohol. On all counts ojas and alcohol are exactly opposite. Other factors that decrease ojas are low or irregular digestion, ama in the body, improper diet and too much exercise.

Not only is what you eat important but how you eat it is important for the production of ojas. Food taken in an atmosphere of congeniality increases ojas.

For other factors that increase ojas, see the chapter on emotions.

Vegetarian Diet

Although it is not necessary to be a vegetarian to enjoy the benefits of the Maharishi Vedic Medicine, a vegetarian diet is recommended because there are many advantages to not eating meat. Obesity, gall bladder disease, hypertension and adult diabetes are found less often in those following a vegetarian diet. Also, vegetarians generally have lower cholesterol, which is a major risk factor in the development of cardiovascular disease.

Whatever foods you eat, it's important not to strain. Enjoy your food and eat more of the foods you know are healthy.

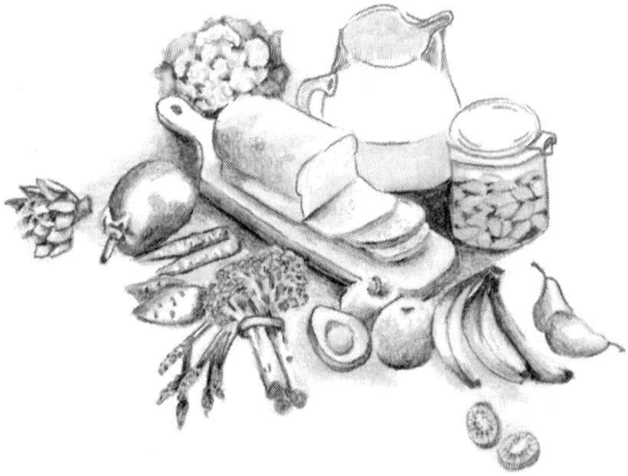

Eat wholesome, organic foods.

Treat Yourself Wisely

Some people eat to live, and others live to eat. Whichever way you look at it, what you eat is very important to your health at every age. If you have been eating foolishly or emotionally, now is the time to treat yourself wisely. Of course, these dietary guidelines are for those who are not under a specific diet recommended by their physician for certain health problems.

References

1. Office of the U.S. Surgeon General 1988. *Surgeon General's report on Nutrition and Health.*
2. Carper, J. 1988. *The Food Pharmacy.* New York: Bantam.
3. Profet, M. 1992. Pregnancy sickness as adaptation: a deterrent to maternal ingestion of teratogens. In Barkow, J.H., Cosmides. L. Tooby, J. (eds). *The Adapted Mind.* New York: Oxford University Press, pp. 327–366.

Chapter Eight

Moderate Exercise, Walking and Maharishi Yoga Asanas

Both Western medicine and Maharishi Vedic Medicine agree, the benefits of exercise are many. What they don't agree on is the amount of exercise, and what type of exercise is right for you specifically.

Weight gain, stiffness, depression and a host of other problems that seem to suddenly appear at menopause can be eliminated through the exercise that is proper for your individual body type.

When Cindy came to see me she was overdoing it on her exercise—jogging, weight lifting and aerobics—three or four times a week. She told me that even though she felt she was doing the "right thing" in relation to exercise, she actually felt tired rather than energized after her workouts. And, no wonder—she was straining at her exercise regimen instead of enjoying it. When Cindy switched to a program of Maharishi Yoga asanas and walking she felt more relaxed and rejuvenated at the same time. She told me, "I never realized how stretching and letting myself go inward with the Maharishi Yoga asanas would help keep me fit. Instead of dreading my exercise program, I look forward to it. Even better, I can practice it anywhere. I feel as if my whole spine has stretched and I feel as if I have a more youthful walk because of it."

What type of exercise you do depends on your mind-body makeup. Someone with a predominance of Kapha in the physiology will have to exercise more, but, unfortunately, likes to exercise the least. The good news for this type of woman is that when she finally makes up her mind to get into a good exercise routine, nothing will stop her from doing it. Kapha types have great stamina and patience and need to realize that exercise is a great way to get rid of the depression that can come with too much body weight.

A thin Vata-type of woman may not like to get into an exercise routine because she's never had to exercise to maintain a low body weight. But she is also susceptible to rapid bone loss at menopause. Bone loss can be reduced through bone-building exercise. Pitta types need to learn not to over exercise, which can cause a build-up of ama in the physiology.

Individual Differences

If you have been exercising vigorously, menopause is a good time to ease up a little. If you haven't been exercising regularly, if at all, menopause marks a good time to change that neglectful lifestyle and start exercising. Regular exercise, approximately half an hour of exercise daily, is the minimum and maximum requirement. The main reason for this is that Vata dosha dominates more with age and exercise increases Vata dosha, which governs movement in the body. When you increase Vata dosha, everything moves along with it.

You also have to look at your predominant dosha. Exercise decreases Kapha dosha, which is in charge of weight. Therefore, those with a predominance of Kapha dosha need more vigorous exercise in order to reduce Kapha in the physiology and avoid sluggishness and weight gain. The Pitta-type woman needs moderate exercise to help her blow off steam and keep healthy, whereas the Vata-type woman should have mild, daily exercise to avoid fatigue, but not so much that she becomes thinner. Therefore, it is the *quality* of the exercise you do in the half hour you allow yourself, not the quantity.

The Benefits of Exercise

Many studies show that exercise improves general fitness and controls illness such as hypertension and diabetes. It strengthens the muscles and cardiovascular system. People who exercise are more likely to lose weight compared with non-exercisers.[1] Those who exercise have more optimal waist-to-hip ratios and a lower incidence of diabetes and coronary experiences, even if overweight.[2] Regular exercise also prevents excessive loss of lean body mass. Moreover, regular exercise has been shown to have a beneficial effect on flexibility, coordination, mood and alertness.[3]

However, there simply are not that many people out there who exercise on a regular basis. The Center for Disease Control and Prevention found that low recreational activity was strongly related to major weight gain during each preceding ten-year period. Of adults who do exercise, only 22% currently exercise at a level beneficial for cardiovascular fitness.[4]

Studies have begun to show more specific benefits of exercise in women. Proper diet plus exercise can produce similar weight loss in the lower and upper body in obese women.[5] Six months after a 12-week program in post-menopausal women, weight was significantly reduced, high-density lipoprotein was still higher and triglycerides still lower. If the women continued to exercise, there was a greater decrease in weight, fat tissue mass, and abdomen-to-total body fat mass compared to the group only on a diet.[6]

The bad news is, compared with men, the evidence is especially strong that although exercise may help maintain lean body mass in women, it is not a significantly useful isolated approach to weight loss.[7] In other words, you were meant to be somewhat padded and, to get that padding off (though not all the way off, which would be unhealthy), you have to eat properly.

It is thought that women have a harder time dropping extra fat due to the effects of estrogen and progesterone receptors on fat cells in women, or due to the need to use less oxygen for a given amount of exercise, or differences in fat distribution.

How Much Exercise Is Enough?

The ancient texts of Ayurveda say that exercise should be practiced daily and in moderation. It is much easier to make exercise a daily habit than a three-times-a-week or every-other-day habit. So what is moderation?

Maharishi Vedic Medicine advises that when you start to sweat profusely, or when breathing begins to be heavy or labored, so that you have to breathe through the mouth, that is the time to stop exercising. If you haven't exercised in a while or are obese, this time may be just a few minutes. It doesn't matter here about the length of time—what matters is having the wisdom to stop. This amount of exercise, which is understood to be 50% of capacity, is balanced and ideal for health. What do I mean by 50% capacity? It means don't exercise to the maximum, which causes stress on the physiology.

Out-of-balance Pitta types will want to jump right in to an exercise program, setting goals and imposing too vigorous exercise routines, thus setting themselves up for failure, and then abandoning exercise altogether. Excessive exercise is not recommended *ever.* In Maharishi Vedic Medicine, to maintain the physiology's overall internal balance is the way to health. Too much exercise can be as harmful (injuries, body aches) as too little. You always must remember that balance, and in the case of exercise, moderation, is the key. Pushing the body near its maximum capacity does strengthen musculature, and may have some benefits in the look of the muscles, but it can cause strain and imbalances in other parts of the body. The system as a whole loses balance, even though some of its parts gain strength.

Because many women gain unwanted weight at menopause, losing weight is a concern. But use better health as your goal and not some unrealistic scale weight. Even less than 10% weight loss improves glycemia control, hypertension, and cholesterol in those with complications of obesity.

Vata types do best with slow-paced, light exercise that keeps the body in motion for fifteen to twenty continuous minutes. They love walking and it is a great exercise for them. Light swimming and easy biking are also recommended. Pitta types naturally have more stamina; so, they can walk, bike and swim, but at a faster pace. They also like to compete, Pitta-types being the movers and shakers of the world, so competitive sports that keep the body in motion for fifteen to twenty continuous minutes is great and enjoyable for them. Recommended exercises are tennis, racquetball, moderate cross-country skiing, biking, swimming, weight lifting, and brisk walking.

Kapha types are definitely recommended to adopt the use of weights. They have the highest capacity and the greatest need to start and stay on a more vigorous exercise program, because it helps them with their weight problems. Vigorous exercise that lasts for fifteen to thirty minutes is best. Recommended exercises for Kapha types are jogging, vigorous biking, swimming, cross-country skiing, heavy weight lifting, aerobics and walking. All types are recommended to practice Maharishi Yoga asanas, which are exercises that promote balance and flexibility. For more information on Maharishi Yoga asanas, contact a Maharishi Ayur-Veda health center listed in the index.

Because your doshic balance is a mixture, Vata/Pitta, Pitta/Kapha, etc., you can integrate the advice for different doshas. For example, a Pitta likes competition and a Kapha needs more vigorous exercise, so a tennis match for a Pitta/Kapha would be good for this type.

The Best Time of Day to Exercise

First, let's look at when exercise is *not* a good idea. Do not exercise when you have an acute illness, or too near meal time, or for at least two hours after a large meal, or for at least one hour after a snack or light meal. After exercise, you should wait at least a half hour before eating.

Maharishi Vedic Medicine considers the morning the best time for physical exercise, the Kapha period from sunrise to 10 a.m. being the optimal time. This is because exercise counteracts the Kapha tendency to be sluggish. The Pitta time of day, between 10 a.m. and 2 p.m., but especially at noon, is not recommended for exercise because you are usually eating your main meal of the day at that time. After 2 p.m. is okay.

A walk after your evening meal is recommended, but not strenuous exercise, as it is too enlivening to be performed so close to bedtime. Evening is the time to wind down, not windup. It is better to spend the evening in more relaxing endeavors, especially for Vata types and for those with sleep problems, which are prevalent at menopause.

You also need to change your exercise at seasonal changes. During the hot summer weather, exercise should be less intense while during the winter, it should definitely not be missed, because it counteracts Kapha.

Walking

Both modern medicine and ancient wisdom agree, walking is one of the best exercises you can do for your health. It is good for any type of physiology. Risk of heart problems in post-menopausal women appears to be greatly decreased by leisure-time physical activity. Even just 30 to 45 minutes of walking three times each week is beneficial.[8] But walking every day is recommended by Maharishi Vedic Medicine.

Walking has an overall beneficial effect of reducing the risk of fracture in osteoporosis. It has a beneficial effect on cardiovascular conditioning and reduces body mass in a beneficial way. These changes, as well as the exercise itself, will improve balance and, in so doing, decrease the risk of falling. In a cross-sectional study, walking was associated with a reduced risk of hip fracture, even when adjusted for bone mineral density, indicating the importance of balance and its effect on falling.[9]

Vata types can be more leisurely with walking, while Kapha types can walk more briskly and for longer periods of time. Those competitive Pitta types should remember that even walking can be overdone. No one should go for long walks in summer's heat or in the chill of winter (which will especially aggravate Vata).

Early morning is a great time to walk because it wakes you up and gets you going. In cold weather walk indoors, or use an exercise machine that especially works the lower part of the body, because more of the overall muscle mass is located there.

Overall, exercises that involve continuous movement, such as walking or biking, are better for you than the stop-and-start sports like tennis or baseball.

Maharishi Yoga Asanas

Like Cindy, many of my patients tell me how much they enjoy the flexibility they feel when they regularly perform Maharishi Yoga asanas. They are easy to do at any age and can be done anywhere without equipment.

Maharishi Yoga asanas are exercises that not only strengthen the muscles and cardiovascular system, but also make your body flexible and integrate mind and body coordination. They are called Maharishi Yoga asanas to differentiate them from some of the more "modern" yoga techniques—such as power yoga, which deviates from the traditional yoga postures and is not in the ancient Ayurvedic texts. Maharishi Yoga asanas are mentioned here because of their known value of promoting balance and health.

These exercises are from a part of Vedic Medicine called *yoga*. The word "yoga" means "union" or "integration," and the exercises are designed to produce integration of mind and body. The word "asana" refers to any of the yoga postures. There is another component to these practices call *pranayama*, or breathing exercises which regulate the breath. Practicing pranayama helps balance the nervous system and breathing, and also integrates mind and body.

This combination of Maharishi Yoga asanas and pranayama will settle the mind and enliven the body. Also, one of the big benefits of practicing asanas is that it relieves stiffness, especially in the neck, back, and shoulders, which is a Vata complaint. Regular practice of Maharishi Yoga asanas helps prevent the rigidity of the musculoskeletal system that is a sign of aging.

Maharishi Yoga asanas massage the inner organs by enlivening the *marmas*, 108 vital points in the body just beneath the skin. The marmas are considered to be connecting points between mind and body. Specific marmas influence specific organ systems; so each yoga posture, by enlivening certain marmas, affects certain organs. Enlivening marmas also increases balance throughout the body.

Studies show that those who practice asanas maintain a flexible physiology that is characteristic of a youthful body. They also have found that they relieve anxiety and tension, decrease mental fatigue, improve memory, reduce serum cholesterol level, increase resistance to physical stress, decrease resting heart rate, reduce blood cholesterol level and are responsible for a host of other improvements.[10, 11]

You should add these exercises into your daily routine of walking and other forms of exercise. However, some women do only Maharishi Yoga asanas and walking and this keeps them trim, healthy, and flexible in both mind and body.

Weight-bearing exercise is recommended to help with prevention of osteoporosis. One of the most popular Maharishi Yoga asanas, *Surya Namaskar*, or the "sun salute," which integrates the whole physiology is also considered a weight-bearing exercise—as the weight you bear is your own.

The sun salute integrates all the major muscle groups. It's a great basic exercise, done slowly and easily. Unfortunately, some celebrities have demonstrated this exercise on television, and have added some incorrect methods of performing the exercise. An instructor trained in Maharishi Yoga asanas can show you how to properly practice this technique.

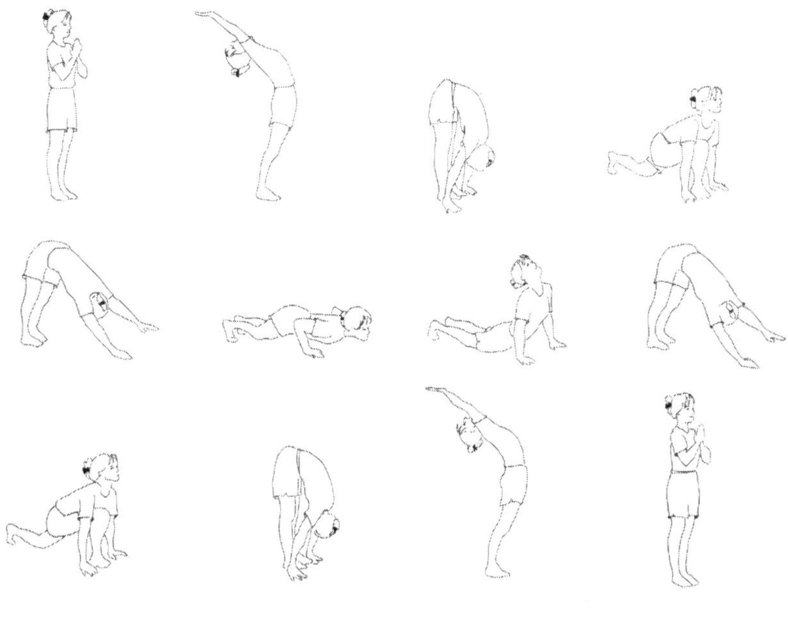

The twelve positions of the sun salute.

Maharishi Vedic Medicine's guidelines on exercise

- In general, exercise to 50 percent of your capacity. For example, if you can swim twelve laps at most, stop after six.
- Exercise every day unless you are ill.
- Don't exercise on a full stomach—wait two hours after a full meal. Also, after you finish exercising, wait half an hour before eating again.
- Do not strain when you exercise. If you start to breathe heavily through the mouth or start perspiring, cut back for now and then gradually increase the amount of exercise. If you feel invigorated, not fatigued, at the end of your exercise period, you are doing the right amount.
- Exercise during the Kapha cycle in the morning (6 a.m. to 10 a.m.) for the best results. The best time to do most exercises is just after your practice of the Transcendental Meditation technique (except for your Maharishi Yoga asanas, which are ideal for settling the mind and body before practicing the TM technique).
- The correct amount and intensity of exercise depends on age: those under 25 need the most, those over 40 need to be more moderate. It also depends on the predominant dosha:

    Vata: Slow-paced, light exercise that keeps the body in motion for 15 to 20 continuous minutes is best. Suggested exercises include walking, swimming, Maharishi Yoga asanas and light bicycling.

    Pitta: Brisker-paced but moderate exercise that keeps your body in motion for 15 to 20 continuous minutes is best. Suggested exercises include brisk walking, moderate cross-country skiing, swimming, cycling, weight lifting, tennis and racquetball.

    Kapha: Vigorous exercise that lasts for 15 to 30 minutes is best. Suggested exercises include jogging, vigorous bicycling, swimming, cross-country skiing, aerobic workouts, walking and heavy weight lifting.

    Exercises for all three doshas: Walking and Maharishi Yoga asanas. You can vary the speed and intensity of your walk according to the predominant dosha. Kaphas may prefer jogging or aerobic walking, while Vatas may prefer a continuous stroll.

These are only suggestions; you should not feel restricted to this list.

Pranayama

The ancient texts say that these breathing techniques create balance in the physiology, improve nervous system functioning and benefit many specific organs. These techniques create refinement in the body by working on Vata dosha. Since Vata dosha is in charge of movement and leads the other two doshas, pranayama

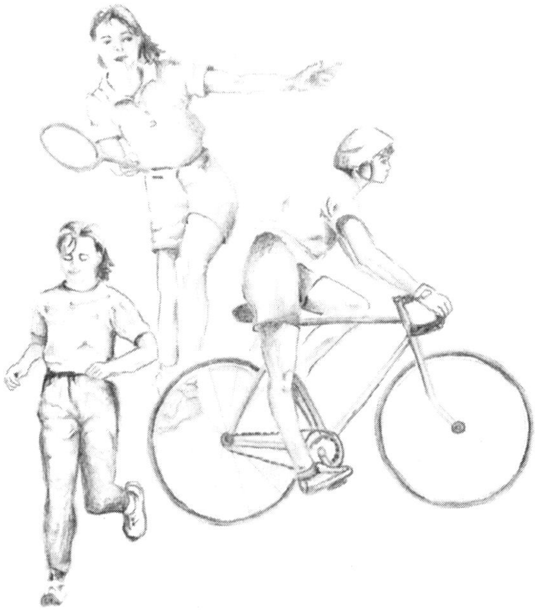

Choose the activity appropriate for your body type.

settles, balances, and refreshes the whole body.

Modern research has found that the practice of pranayama: reduces bronchial asthma attacks,[12] increases breath-holding capacity and lowers pulse rate.[13]

Pranayama should be practiced twice a day for five minutes following exercise and/or Maharishi Yoga asanas, but before the Transcendental Meditation technique. An instructor of Maharishi Yoga asanas can show you the proper breathing techniques.

The Three Parts of Exercise in Maharishi Vedic Medicine

Maharishi Vedic Medicine works on three levels: the body, the breath, and the mind. Each morning you begin with exercising the body by performing the sun salute, or other asanas, which have been given to you by a qualified practitioner of Maharishi Vedic Medicine. Next are the breathing techniques of pranayama for the breath, and then the practice of the Transcendental Meditation technique for the mind.

Do these things daily and you will keep flexible, stimulate your organs, and prevent the stiffness, sluggishness, and weight problems that can come at menopause. On top of all that, you keep your mind and body integrated and balanced. Do not neglect yourself in this area. (See Questions and Answers for more information on Maharishi yoga asanas.)

References

1. National Institutes of Health Consensus Development Conference statement. 1985. Health implications of obesity. *Ann Intern Med*, 103,1073.
2. Blair, S.N.1993. Evidence for success of exercise in weight loss and control. *Ann Intern Med* 1, 19, 702.
3. Exercise in the postmenopausal woman. 1987. Bachmann, G.A., Grill, J. *Geriatrics*, January, 42, 1, 75-7, 81-5.
4. *Women's Health Source Book III*, p. 332.
5. Kanaley, J.A., Andresen-Reid, M.L., Oenning. L. et al.1993. Differential health benefits of weight loss in upper-body and lower-body obese women. *American Journal of Clinical Nutrition*, 57, 20.
6. Svendsen, O.L., Hassager. C. & Christiansen, C. 1994. Six months' follow-up on exercise added to a short-term diet in overweight post-menopausal women—effects on body composition, resting metabolic rate, cardiovascular risk factors and bone. *Int J Obes Relat Metab Disord*, 18, 692.
7. Gleim, G.W. 1993. Exercise is not an effective weight loss modality in women. *Journal of American Coll Nutr*, 12, 363.
8. Lemaitre, R.N., Heckbert, S.R., Psaty, B.M., et al. 1995. Leisure-time physical activity and the risk of non-fatal myocardial infarction in post-menopausal women. *Arch Intern Med.*, 155, 2302.
9. Cummings, et al. 1995. *New England Journal of Medicine*, 332, 767.
10. Udupa, K.N., Singh, R.H. & Yadava, R.A. 1975b. Psychological

and biochemical responses to the practice of Hatha Yoga in young normal volunteers. *Indian Journal of Medical Research* 61(2), 237–244.

11. Santha, J.K., Sridharan, S.K., Patil, M.L., 1981. Physiological and biochemical parameters in subjects undergoing yogic training. *Indian Journal of Medical Research,* 75, 120–124.
12. Bhole, M.V. 1967. Treatment of bronchial asthma by yogic methods. *Yoga Mimansa,* 9(3), 33–41.
13. Nayar, H.S., Mathur, R.M., Sampath, K.R. 1995. Effects of yogic exercises on human physical efficiency. *Indian Journal of Medical Research,* 63 (1), 1369–1376.

CHAPTER NINE

Handling Hot Flashes, Preventing Bone Loss, and Cardiovascular Problems

Prior to natural menopause, menopause-related changes begin. This is the menopause transition or "perimenopause." The perimenopausal years are a time of many changes. Fluctuations in the levels of hormones produced by the ovaries lead to normal, short-term physical changes, such as irregular menstrual patterns and hot flashes. Long-term changes carry an increased risk of osteoporosis and heart disease.

Other changes associated with perimenopause and menopause include night sweats, fatigue, mood swings, vaginal dryness, fluctuations in sexual desire or response, forgetfulness and difficulty sleeping. Depression, headaches, dizziness, and heart palpitations have not been proven by Western science to be related to menopause, but they can be concerns at this time. All of these changes are related to imbalances in Vata, Pitta or Kapha doshas in some way.

Although there is a wide range of possible menopause-related conditions, most women going through natural menopause have minimal disturbances during the perimenopausal years. With proper attention to diet, exercise and daily routine, many disturbances diminish or disappear over time.

Hot Flashes

Leslee, age 42, had a hysterectomy three years prior to seeing me and she still had her ovaries. She was having extreme hot flashes combined with extreme anxiety and anger. She said, "I get angry very easily and I cry a lot. I can't concentrate. I hate myself. I'm just so sad."

Low estrogen levels are linked to some uncomfortable symptoms in many women. The most common and easy to recognize symptom is hot flashes—sudden intense waves of heat and sweating. They usually last between three and six minutes and may occur up to several times a day. Some women find that these hot flashes disrupt their sleep, and others report mood changes that could be due to lack of sleep.

Hot flashes, also known as vasomotor flushes, are experienced by many women within three years of menopause.[1] However, some women don't experience them at all. Hot flashes are characterized by a feeling of heat and sweating, usually involving the head and neck to a great degree. At night, a woman may throw off her blankets, soak the sheets with sweat, then feel cold a few minutes later and need even more blankets. Skin surface temperature increases during a hot flash. Some women experience these for a few months, for some they last a few years, and for a rare group of women, they go on for a decade or more.

Hot flashes are thought by Western medicine to be related to norepinephrine metabolism in the brain, related to estrogen deprivation. Norepinephrine is a neurotransmitter, one of those peptides that sends messages from our brains to our organs and immune system, which the system sends to the brain.

Because hot flashes involve the neuroendocrine system, stress tends to increase them. Not all hot flashes are related to decreases in estrogen. Hyperthyroidism can cause them, as can alcohol intake and out-of-control diabetes. Some women have hot flashes so continually that they result in sleep deprivation, particularly in interruption of rapid eye movement (REM) sleep, the type of sleep associated with dreaming. This can result in depression.

In Maharishi Vedic Medicine too much heat in the body is

known to be produced by an imbalance of Pitta dosha. Maharishi Vedic Medicine herbal supplements along with a balanced diet will help relieve symptoms. A physician trained in Maharishi Ayur-Veda may also recommend special foods or drinks that are correct for your constitution and will help with hot flashes.

Leslee was also feeling heat in her abdomen area and had a gassy stomach. She had numbness and tingling in her arms from time to time that made them painful to lift. Along with needed changes in her diet and Maharishi Vedic Medicine prescriptions, came some specific herbal recommendations to improve her calcium absorption. She also took herbs to help clear out impurities and to help balance her hormones, emotions, mind, nerves, elimination and blood. I recommended specific aroma therapy to help calm her Pitta and herbal supplements to help uplift her emotions and improve her metabolism. Aloe vera mixed with water in the morning helped both her hot flashes and her digestive problems.

Leslee said, "I am able to cope with stress better and I'm feeling better overall. I'm not getting as angry. Concentration is better. There is less anxiety, my arms feel less numb. I am still up and down emotionally and I would like to feel, physically, more energy." At this point she learned the TM technique, and in the following months she felt much more emotional stability. The numbness and tingling went away completely. She felt a deeper connection with herself and felt that many positive changes were happening in her life.

I advised her to continue having seasonal follow-ups and I also advised her to have Maharishi rejuvenation and purification treatments. Even though Leslee came to see me mainly for her extreme hot flashes and anger she is the type of woman who could have ended up having to seek psychiatric treatments because of all of her related emotional problems. By treating her in the comprehensive approach of Maharishi Vedic Medicine, she was able to grasp the knowledge and wisdom of Maharishi Ayur-Veda. Being an insightful person, she was able to connect to herself and address her problems at a deeper level.

Osteoporosis

Hormones are necessary for regulation of bone metabolism. When the body stops producing these hormones, some women may end up with osteoporosis due to increased Vata, which results in accelerated bone loss after menopause. This is particularly true of thinner-boned Vata and Pitta types. However, the rate of loss slowly lessens as a woman ages. At the age of 70 or older, women parallel the loss that males experience. At all ages, however, women will have lower bone mineral densities than men. According to the National Osteoporosis Foundation, women are four times more likely than men to develop the disease.

Nanette had great concerns about her bone density because of a strong family history of osteoporosis. She had a bone density scan done and was within the normal range for her age, but because of her family history had been advised by her gynecologist to take medication to increase bone density.

Osteoporosis is the loss of bone mass, most often seen in midlife, that causes bones to become gradually weaker, thinner, and more brittle. The *American Journal of Medicine* defines osteoporosis as "a systemic skeletal disease characterized by low bone mass and microarchitectural deterioration of bone tissue with a consequent increase in bone fragility and susceptibility to fracture."[2] The first sign of osteoporosis is often a broken bone.

"Among the most eye-opening data is that osteoporosis is more costly and more common than cardiovascular disease," said Robin Foust, director of program development at Health Management Corporation, a Richmond, Virginia-based wellness consulting firm.[2]

An out-of-balance Vata-type woman fits the profile of those most susceptible to osteoporosis. The key phrase here is *out of balance.* Those who live on soft drinks, caffeine, and who don't exercise regularly are especially susceptible. A study undertaken at the Grand Forks Human Nutrition Research Center on people who drank sodas regularly and did not eat a healthy diet consisting of leafy greens and whole grains, found that the sugary sodas robbed the bones of phosphorus. Phosphorus was measured because it's a major bone mineral that also supplies energy to the cells. Sodas are not only packed with "empty" calories, but they rob the body of nutrients.

Nanette was a petite woman with a lot going on in her physiology besides the fear of osteoporosis. She was extremely anxious, tired, had hot flashes and had been put on hormone replacement therapy that caused excessive hair loss and gave her constant headaches, so she stopped taking it. She also had lower back pain, seasonal allergies and a thyroid nodule which was hyperactive. She had had a partial thyroidectomy and was treated with radioactive iodine. Besides her other medications she was on Synthyroid, a thyroid medication.

She also had irregular bowel movements with constipation, cramping in her legs, as well as her toes, and she didn't sleep through the night. She was also experiencing ringing in the ears.

I mention all of her other problems here because rarely does a woman come to me with one problem. And actually, osteoporosis wasn't a problem with Nanette, but she was told it *could* be a problem, which she worried about above everything else. But what I am underscoring here is that it is a common finding in Maharishi Vedic Medicine that when you treat the problems from the source, everything improves.

For Nanette, the first thing she noticed during her first month of treatment was that she started having a bowel movement every day. Proper elimination is the key to getting rid of toxic build-up in the body. Her energy level went up and her hot flashes went down. Her headaches came down dramatically from having one once a day to having one once a week.

The following month she started sleeping better and her headaches were virtually gone except for an occasional one. She was still concerned with the hair loss and ringing in her ears but she was experiencing greater health in all areas.

She decided to learn the TM technique. During this time she had a thyroid test and realized that she needed only half the dose of thyroid medication, which surprised her as well as her primary care physician. After this she said that almost everything had improved and that her hair loss was much less.

Reduced Cardiovascular Risk Factor

Research published in American Heart Association journals *Stroke and Hypertension* shows that the Transcendental Meditation program:

- Significantly reduces blockage of blood vessels supplying blood to the brain and the heart without change in diet or exercise. These results correlated with a 11% reduction in risk of heart attack due to atherosclerosis, and a 7.7–15% reduction in risk of stroke due to atherosclerosis.
- Is twice as effective as other relaxation techniques in reducing hypertension without change in diet or exercise. These results correlated with a 35–40% reduction in risk of stroke due to hypertension and a 20–45% reduction in risk of coronary heart disease due to hypertension.
- Produces a 15% reduction in lipid peroxide (cholesterol) levels, associated with reduced risk for atherosclerosis.

References: 1. A. Castillo-Richmond, M.D. et al., "Effects of Stress Reduction on Cartoid Atherosclerosis in Hypertensive African Americans," *Stroke*, vol. 31 (2000), pp. 568–573.

2. R.H. Schneider, M.D. et al., "A Randomized Controlled Trial of Stress Reduction for Hypertension in Older African Americans," *Hypertension*, vol. 26 (1995), pp. 820–827.

3. C.N. Alexander et al., "A Trial of Stress Reduction for Hypertension in Older African Americans (Part II): Gender and Risk Subgroup Analysis," *Hypertension*, vol. 28 (1996), pp. 228–237.

4. R.H. Schneider, M.D. et al., "Lower Lipid Peroxide Levels in Practitioners of the *Transcendental Meditation* Program," *Psychosomatic Medicine*, vol. 60 (1998), pp. 38–41.

Many endocrine problems, like thyroid (which in conventional medicine usually does not get better by itself) can be improved with Maharishi Ayur-Veda treatments. In this case no attention was really put on her thyroid problem although there are special herbs and herbal preparations in Ayur-Veda for thyroid problems. The overall corrections to the imbalances, bringing improved health to the whole mind and body with the TM technique and other Maharishi Vedic Medicine therapies, caused positive changes in all areas.

Nanette then had a follow-up with her gynecologist and she was recommended to go back on hormones and medication for bone density. After her own research and a lot of thinking, Nanette decided to stay with Maharishi Vedic Medicine to address her menopausal concerns and to have a healthy menopause in a natural way. I recommended several foods to her that are rich in calcium, especially green leafy vegetables, Maharishi Amrit Kalash™ herbal supplements, a specific natural calcium supplement and other Maharishi Vedic Medicine herbal compounds. To prevent problems with osteoporosis she was recommended to continue practicing Maharishi Yoga asanas, brisk walking and warm oil self-massage. For further rejuvenation I told her to go on a regular basis (at least twice a year) to a Maharishi Ayur-Veda Health Center. She later told me that she did go for a week of treatments and not only did she feel wonderful but the final problem—cramping in her toes—had gone away.

LuAnn, a Kapha-type woman, came to see me because she was in menopause and her bone density scan indicated bone of two standard deviations below normal range. She was on natural progesterone and high doses of calcium. She had been put on Raloxifene by her family physician but had developed extreme nausea and hair loss. When she was put on a lesser dosage, the nausea still occurred along with digestive problems. She had a long-standing case of hemorrhoids that was currently bothering her.

Even though LuAnn was taking natural progesterone, she was still having a few hot flashes during the day, seasonal allergies, and post nasal drip during fall and winter. She also wanted to lose some weight.

Taking a calcium supplement doesn't always work if the calcium isn't absorbed. So, to improve LuAnn's calcium absorption and rebuild her bones, I recommended a natural dietary supplement which aids calcium absorption. Most of her symptoms were Kapha-related, so she started a Kapha-balancing diet. Adding more green leafy vegetables to her diet also helped her receive the nutrients she needed without adding unwanted calories. The proper exercise, daily oil self-massage, and special herbal supplements greatly uplifted her mood. The bigger-boned Kapha-type woman can be susceptible to osteoporosis because of an imbalance in the first level of the dhatus—rasa dhatu, which is the principle upholding the first products of digested food. If the digestion is not working properly then all the other dhatus are disturbed: blood, muscle, adipose tissue, bone, nervous system and ovum. For health on *all* levels, the first level must be working properly.

Protein Consumption and Bone Fractures

Maharishi Vedic Medicine favors a healthy, vitamin- and mineral-rich, organic vegetarian diet. Some studies have shown that dietary protein increases urinary calcium losses and have been associated with higher rates of hip fracture. Protein was associated with an increased risk of forearm fracture for women who consumed more than 95 grams of protein supplements per day compared with those who consumed less than 68 grams per day. A similar increase in risk was observed with ingestion of animal protein, but no association was found for consumption of vegetable protein. Women who consumed five or more servings of red meat per week also had a significantly increased risk of forearm fracture compared with women who ate red meat less than once per week.[3]

Exercise and Natural Calcium

Diet is extremely important. Low calcium diets or very large intakes of caffeine and alcohol are all associated with osteoporosis. To help prevent excess bone loss—a calcium-rich diet, weight-bearing exercise (especially sun salutations), walking and Maharishi Ayur-Veda purification and rejuvenation programs are all recommended.

Smoking and a sedentary lifestyle also increase risk of bone loss. Exercise can increase bone mass. Thirty minutes of exercise a day is good for your overall physiology, especially bone density. Walking is excellent. Weight lifting should be performed with caution if osteoporosis is advanced. Gentle Maharishi Yoga asanas should be performed slowly and with care.

Calcium is also recommended, but from natural sources rather than synthetic. Natural sources are sesame seeds, sunflower seeds, almonds, soybeans, soy milk and its products, cow's milk and its products, carrots, coconut, almond milk, broccoli, green leafy vegetables and certain shells.

Literally thousands of articles have been written about the average daily requirement of calcium for women of various ages. A consensus by Western medical standards suggests that women on hormone replacement therapy should also ingest 1,000 mg of calcium per day, and women not on HRT should ingest 1,500 mg of calcium per day.[4]

Chewing a handful of sesame seeds in the morning each day provides natural calcium. (A note of caution for women with hot flashes—sesame seeds are heating.) Natural Maharishi Ayur-Veda herbal formulas of calcium, magnesium and zinc are also recommended. Ten minutes of exposure to sunlight a day will help the the body create vitamin D, which is good for flexible, strong bones. Any more than ten minutes of direct exposure is not recommended, due to the sun's harmful effects on the skin. To monitor your bone density a DEXA (duel energy X-ray absorptiometry) scan may be advised, especially if you have a family history of osteoporosis.

The ancient Ayurvedic texts recognized bone loss as a problem even thousands of years ago. The texts highly recommend a daily warm oil self-massage to help keep the bones flexible. A daily warm oil self-massage also calms and balances the emotions.

After one month of treatment LuAnn felt that her digestion and energy had both improved. She did not have any more problems with hemorrhoids and her congestion and post nasal drip were better. I advised her to have regular follow-ups and bone density scans on a regular basis. By following the total program she feels more vital, with no adverse side effects, and she is pleased that she can comply with the program because of its ease.

It is important to note that there are several Ayurvedic herbs and minerals which help increase bone density, reduce osteoporosis and fractures. Ask your physician trained in Maharishi Ayur-Veda for specific recommendations.

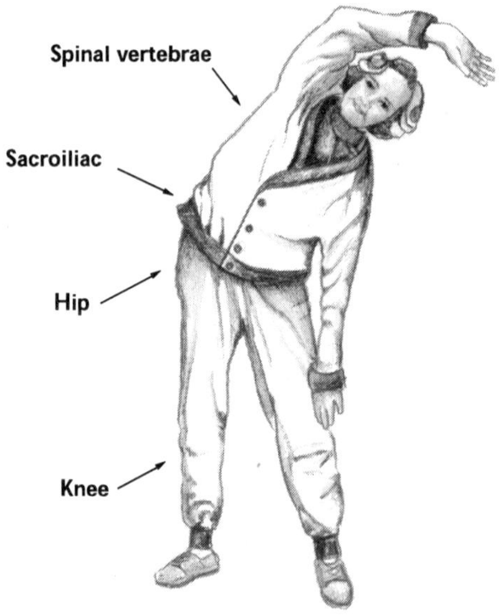

Osteoarthritis most commonly affects the knee joint, hip joint, sacroiliac, and spinal vertebrae.

Heart Disease

Just as many women have a negative association with menopause because it is a sign of aging, many women think that heart disease can only happen in old age and can be dealt with "later."

Women take it for granted that heart disease won't happen to them. In fact, heart disease is the leading killer of women in the United States and is spreading to other industrialized countries.

Statistics show that one out of every two women in the U.S. will eventually die of heart disease. One half million women die each year from cardiovascular disease, including stroke and congestive heart failure. Of those, 250,000 die from heart attacks. Twice as many women die from heart disease and stroke as from all cancers.[5]

Heart disease, which is known scientifically as coronary heart disease, occurs when the heart sustains damage due to narrowed or blocked arteries within the organ. Such blockages make it impossible for blood to reach the heart muscle. The most dramatic and potentially life-threatening result of this process is a heart attack, also known as acute myocardial infarction. The chest discomfort known as angina pectoris is a warning that the blood supply to the heart is insufficient.

Even though women account for almost half of heart attack deaths, they are unlikely to believe they're at risk of cardiovascular disease. When women were asked what they think is the leading cause of mortality, they say breast cancer. It's not. It's coronary disease.[6] Of course, not all women who have heart attacks are in menopause, but most women who have heart attacks are menopausal.

The statistics (based on the United States) are:[7]

- 93,000 women die each year in the United States of stroke, whereas breast cancer kills 43,600 women
- At older ages, women who have heart attacks are twice as likely as men to die from them within a few weeks.
- 44 percent of women and 27 percent of men die within one year of a heart attack.
- 480,000 heart attack deaths occur in the United States each year—236,000 victims are women.
- 498,000 women die each year of cardiovascular disease. All forms of cancer combined kill 254,000 women each year.

- In 63 percent of women and 48 percent of men who died suddenly of coronary heart disease, there were no previous symptoms of the disease.
- Smoking has a more dramatic impact on a woman's heart disease risk due to her smaller vessel lumens.
- Hypertension is the most constant risk factor for cardiovascular disease in women over 35.
- Hypertension combined with obesity, plus oral contraceptive use at least doubles cardiovascular disease risk.

Counteracting Stress and Heart Disease

Ayurveda's ancient wisdom notes that a stressful life with no stress management technique is a major factor in poor heart condition. The ancient texts say that one who wishes to protect the heart and circulatory system should avoid, above all else, those causes leading to mental stress and instability.

Hundreds of studies show that the TM technique is the most highly effective stress-reduction technique. One study on hypertension (abnormally high blood pressure) showed that the group of subjects who practiced the TM technique had the greatest reduction of blood pressure and stress, while one of the other relaxation techniques, designed to mimic the TM technique, had worse outcomes than even the control group.[8] Another study showed that the TM technique reduced hypertension more than twice as much as progressive relaxation.[9] The American Heart Association's journal *Stroke* reported that the practice of the TM technique can decrease the risk of stroke and heart attack by reducing the thickness of clogged artery walls.[10]

Because the TM technique has no adverse side effects, any woman can use it. In modern medicine, on the other hand, the drugs prescribed for heart conditions can make matters worse. It is a fact that the adverse side effects from drugs are becoming more predominant than the health benefits of drugs.

This is why in addition to corrections in diet and moderate exercise techniques, the Transcendental Meditation technique is always recommended to relieve the heart of stress.

It is important to note that in my practice all the various aspects of heart disease (for example, hypertensive heart disease, ischemic heart disease, atherosclerotic heart disease, etc.) are treatable with Maharishi Vedic Medicine. These results are very good with no side effects. One of the advantages of Maharishi Vedic Medicine treatment is improvement in the symptoms along with the rejuvenation of the heart and other vital organs (brain, lungs, liver, pancreas, etc.) which receive their blood supply and nutrition from the heart.

There are very specific herbal formulas that help in the treatment of the various forms of heart disease. There are also specific herbal formulas for the heart which can be used on a regular basis to prevent heart disease or to minimize the risk in the early stages of heart disease. I suggest these to some of my patients, especially those who have a family history of heart disease, or those who have any of the other risk factors that can create a disease in the future. You can consult your physician trained in Maharishi Ayur-Veda for the specific recommendations.

References

1. New England Research, Inc.1991 *Women and Their Health in Massachusetts: Final Report 1991.* Watertown, MA: New England Research Institute.
2. Peck, W.A. 1993. Consensus development conference: Diagnosis, prophylaxis, and treatment of osteoporosis. *American Journal of Medicine*, 94, 646.
3. National Institutes of Health. 1991. Osteoporosis: More common than a heart attack. Osteoporosis Research, Education and Health Promotion, National Institute of Arthritis and Musculoskeletal and Skin Diseases. *NIH* Publication.

4. Feskanich, D., Willett, W.C., Stampfer, M.J. & Colditz, G.A.1996 (Mar 1). Protein consumption and bone fractures in women. *American Journal of Epidemiology,* 143(5), 472–479.
5. American Health Consultants. Calcium and osteoporosis. *Women's Health Source Book III,* p. 387.
6, 7. Women's Health Source Book III. *Are women distracted by health threats?* pp. 295–297.
8. Alexander, C.N., Langer E.J., et al., 1989. Transcendental Meditation, mindfulness, and longevity: An experimental study with the elderly. *Journal of Personality and Social Psychology,* 57(6), 950–964.
9. Alexander, C.N., Robinson, P., et al. 1994a. The effect of Transcendental Meditation compared to other methods of relaxation and meditation in reducing risk factors, morbidity, and mortality. *Homeostasis,* 35, 243–264.
10. Castillo-Richmond, A., Schneider, R.H., et al. 2000. Effects of stress reduction and carotid atherosclerosis in hypertensive African Americans. *Stroke,* 31, 568–573.

CHAPTER TEN

Hormones, HRT and Breast Cancer

To briefly review, menopause is the medical term for the end of a woman's menstrual periods. It is a natural part of aging, and occurs when the ovaries start to produce less hormones. This causes estrogen and progesterone levels to drop, and leads to the end of monthly menstrual periods. This usually happens between the ages of 45 and 60, but it can happen earlier. Menopause can also occur when the ovaries are surgically removed or stop functioning for any other reason.

How the Hormones Regulate the Normal Menstrual Period

Before we discuss how the hormonal levels change in menopause, here is a brief understanding of how the hormones regulate the normal menstrual period.

Pre- or perimenopause is not the only time your hormones wildly fluctuate. They also fluctuate at the beginning of menstruation. The major hormones involved in this sign of a maturing woman are Follicle-Stimulating Hormone (FSH) and Luteinizing Hormone (LH), which come from the pituitary gland that is in the brain. Estrogen and progesterone are also major hormones which come from the ovaries. Estrogen is responsible for the changes that take place in girls at puberty: breast enlargement, growth of underarm and pubic hair, pigmentation of the nipples and aureole, and development of the vagina, uterus, and fallopian tubes. The curvy contours of the female body and maturation of the skeleton are all because of estrogen.

Progesterone is the precursor of estrogen and other steroid hormones. It is necessary for the survival of the fertilized ovum, the resulting embryo, and the fetus throughout gestation.

The hypothalamus, located in the brain, produces gonadotrophic-releasing hormones (GnRHs). You can see that the brain and the ovaries are connected.

Hormones are not fluctuating only at the time of perimenopause. As the control messengers for the physiology, hormone levels fluctuate constantly because they are responding to changing bodily needs. The liver is continuously metabolizing and excreting hormones as they pass through the bloodstream.

More about Estrogen

When estrogen was first discovered by researchers, they assumed it was the only fertility-producing hormone. As investigations continued, more types of estrogen were discovered and each was given its own name. Therefore, the word estrogen is the name of the class of hormones that have to do with fertility.[1]

Three main forms of estrogen (from *estrus*, meaning *heat* or *fertility*) occur naturally in your body: estradiol, estrone, and estriol. These three are collectively known as the female sex hormones. They are made primarily in the ovaries but also from androstenedione in fat cells, muscle cells, and skin even after menopause.

Estradiol is the most potent and predominates in premenopausal women. It is 1,000 times more potent in its effects on breast tissue than estriol. Overexposure to estradiol increases the risk of breast cancer.[2]

Estrone is the dominant estrogen after menopause (or postmenopause). It continues to be made by the conversion of the adrenal steroid, androstenediol, primarily in body fat and muscle cells. If there is more fat in the physiology, then more estrone is also there. Some obese women produce more estrogen after menopause than thin premenopausal women.[3]

Estriol is highest during pregnancy. It is made by the placenta from a hormone called DHEA (dehydroepiandrosterone). DHEA and DHEA-S (a sulfated counterpart) are the most abundantly produced hormones in the body. Women with high levels of DHEA-S are known to have less breast cancer and osteoporosis. Interestingly, studies show that those practicing the Transcendental Meditation technique have increased DHEA-S.[4]

Although the word estrogen generally refers to the class of hormones produced by the body, there are also estrogens found outside the body: phytoestrogens, xenoestrogens, natural and synthetic estrogens.

Phytoestrogens refer to plant compounds with estrogen-like activity. They are present in a wide variety of food and herbs and

IMPROVED PHYSICAL HEALTH

Reduced Hospitalization and Doctor's Visits

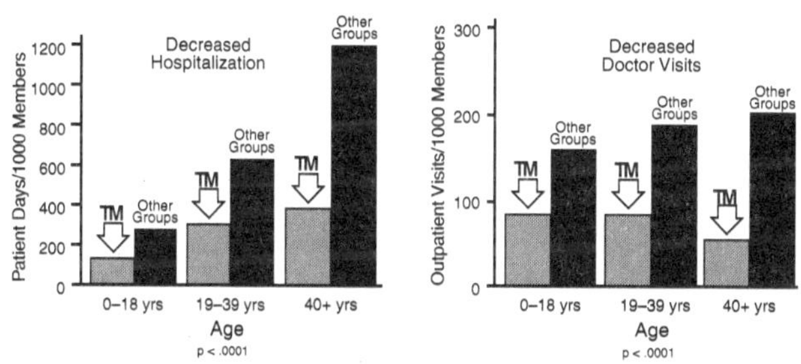

A study of health insurance statistics over a five-year period found that 2000 participants in the Transcendental Meditation program had less than half the doctor visits and hospitalization than other groups of comparable age, gender, profession, and insurance terms. The difference between the groups was greatest for individuals over 40. In addition, the TM program practitioners had markedly fewer incidents of illness in 17 medical treatment categories.

References: 1. D.W. Orme-Johnson, "Medical Care Utilization and the Transcendental Meditation Program," *Psychosomatic Medicine,* 49 (1) (1987), pp. 493-507.
2. D.W. Orme-Johnson and R. Schneider, "Reduced Health Care Utilization in Transcendental Meditation Practitioners," presented at the conference of the Society for Behavioral Medicine (Washington, D.C.), March 22, 1987.

when used in the diet or in specific natural remedies, they can alleviate menopausal symptoms. Examples of phytoestrogens are soy products, cashews, oats, corn, wheat, apples, almonds, lentils, pomegranates and a host of others.

Xenoestrogens, sometimes called environmental estrogens, are considered toxic compounds with estrogen-like activity. Nearly all are petrochemically based. They come from many sources: chemical fertilizers, plastics, drugs and pesticides. We humans made them for the betterment of mankind. But when we tried to improve on Mother Nature, it backfired, and we have ended up polluting ourselves. Xenoestrogens will be discussed more thoroughly in a later chapter. It is a big problem, but one that we women in our wisdom years can tackle, for the sake of future generations.

Natural estrogens are different from phytoestrogens although sometimes the two words are used to mean the same thing. However, the hormone replacement pill known as Premarin is considered a natural estrogen because it comes from a natural source, pregnant mare's urine. It's "natural" but it's not a plant.

Synthetic estrogens made by the pharmaceutical companies are another type of estrogen. These have had their molecular structure altered so they can be patented. A good example of a synthetic estrogen is diethylstilbestrol (DES). DES resembles a phytoestrogen called P-anol, found in fennel and anise plants. It can be inexpensively synthesized and has been used for regulation of the menstrual cycle, in oral contraceptives and to prevent premature labor. The P-anol found in plants is harmless when used in small quantities. But, DES has been implicated in vaginal and cervical cancers in daughters of mothers who were given DES during pregnancy.[5] But DES was also used in beef cattle to fatten them up more quickly because estrogen causes fat buildup.

As you can see, estrogen is not hard to come by.

More about Progesterone

Progesterone is a hormone that is secreted in a woman's body as a response to ovulation in order to ready the uterus for implantation of the egg. It is the primary hormone of fertility and pregnancy and was thus given the name progesterone, meaning "pro-gestation."

If a women skips a period, her body may not be making enough progesterone to break down the uterine lining. By a woman's mid-30's, even though estrogen production may remain adequate while she is still having periods, ovulation rarely occurs. Therefore, estrogen dominance occurs relative to the loss of progesterone. The undesirable effects of too much estrogen in the physiology (breast cancer, uterine fibroids, endometrial cancer, decreased sex drive, fibrocystic breasts) are counteracted by proper levels of progesterone.

During a woman's baby-making years, the follicles, which are the eggs encased in sacs, are stimulated by FSH and produce estrogen. Estrogen levels rise, which signals the hypothalamus to secrete LH-releasing hormone. This signals the pituitary to stop the FSH and to produce a surge of LH. When LH peaks, the body releases an egg from the follicle. This is called ovulation.

Next the follicle, which in this stage is called the *corpus luteum* (it means "yellowish body," so named because of its appearance as a small yellow body, on the surface of the ovary), starts to produce progesterone in addition to estrogen.

These hormones build up the lining of the uterus. Having served its purpose, hormone production levels off. When hormones in the blood drops, the uterus lining is shed, which appears as the menstrual period. When the hypothalamus gets the signal that estrogen and progesterone levels are low, it stimulates FSH and the cycle begins again.

There can be variations to this cycle. If a woman is too thin or has the build of an athlete who is muscular yet has very low fat, the period may not come. When the level of fat increases, the cycle corrects itself and the periods return. The body must be in balance in order to function properly.

Progesterone builds bone and protects against osteoporosis and some types of cancer. It helps normalize blood sugar levels, helps use fat for energy, normalizes zinc and copper levels, is a natural diuretic and, as mentioned before, is necessary for the survival of the embryo and fetus throughout gestation. Progesterone levels at menopause fall by a greater percentage than estrogen levels.

How Hormonal Levels Change in Menopause

For reasons unknown to modern science, the ovaries begin to decline in hormone production during the mid-thirties. In the late forties, the process accelerates and hormones fluctuate more, causing irregular menstrual cycles and unpredictable episodes of heavy bleeding. By the early to mid-fifties, usually around age 51, periods finally end altogether.

However, estrogen production does not completely stop. The ovaries decrease their output significantly, but still may produce a small amount. Also, estrone is produced in fat tissue with help from the adrenal glands. Although this form of estrogen is weaker than that produced by the ovaries, it increases with age and with the amount of fat tissue.

At menopause, hormone levels don't always decline uniformly. During perimenopause, which can be up to six years before your periods finally stop, estrogen levels start to fluctuate. Sometimes your estrogen levels are low, resulting in hot flashes. Sometimes your progesterone is low and your estrogen is high, resulting in PMS-type symptoms.

Changing ovarian hormone levels affect the other glands in the body, which together make up the endocrine system. The endocrine system controls growth, metabolism and reproduction. This system must constantly readjust to work effectively. Ovarian hormones also affect all other tissues, including those of the breasts, vagina, bones, blood vessels, gastrointestinal tract, urinary tract, and skin.

As mentioned earlier, many cultures do not consider menopause a disease or a health problem. A study by Dr. Peter Ellison at Harvard University on ovarian hormone levels in various populations noted that premenopausal estrogen levels in Western women are so high that they should be considered abnormal. High hormone levels found in Western cultures were thought to be a reflection of lack of exercise combined with overeating.[6]

Dr. John R. Lee, in his book *What Your Doctor May Not Tell You About Menopause*, notes that "Ellison suggests the higher ovarian function common in Western populations results in a proportionately greater fall in hormone levels at menopause, and this may account for the greater incidence and severity of menopausal symptoms seen. In non-industrialized populations, the discrepancy between pre- and post-menopausal hormone levels is considerably less than in industrialized populations. Remember, post-menopausal estrogen levels do not drop to zero, they merely drop to the level that will not produce a blood-rich uterine lining to be shed. If Dr. Ellison's hypothesis is correct, it may mean that prevention of menopausal symptoms could be accomplished by eating less and getting more exercise."[7]

Hormone Replacement Therapy

The combination therapy of estrogen plus progesterone is called hormone replacement therapy (HRT). HRT is the most widely prescribed drug for women who are experiencing menopausal symptoms. At menopause, every woman should weigh the personal risks against the benefits of HRT. A famous study began in 1996 when almost 122,000 female registered nurses, ages 30–55, were enrolled to analyze mortality related to hormone replacement therapy, with a focus on cardiovascular disease and cancer deaths. A questionnaire was used every two years to track informa-

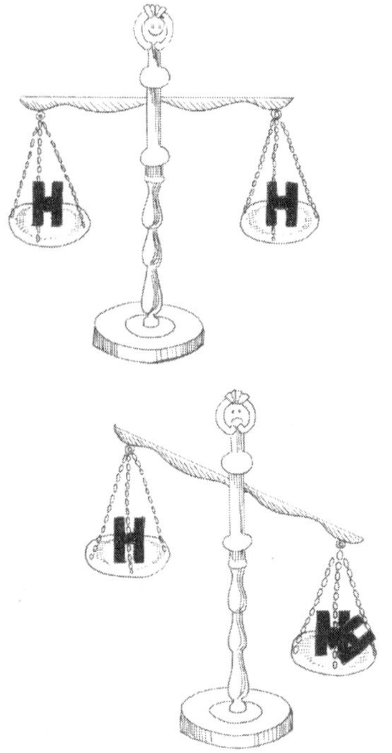

Fluctuating hormones can create imbalance in the physiology. Maharishi Vedic Medicine helps restore balance.

tion on risk factors, HRT status, and any new diagnosis of significant illness or death.

Almost all of the statistics about HRT—both pro and con—come from this study. Although many of the statistics support use of HRT as beneficial for those at risk for coronary artery disease and osteoporosis, there was an increase in breast cancer. In the words of some of the latest research on HRT, "The complexity in weighing the risks and benefits arises because the benefits of long-term therapy are offset by a 43 percent higher risk of dying from breast cancer after 10 years. Partly due to these risks for breast cancer, the life-preserving benefits of estrogen appear to decrease after 10 years of use."[8]

There are known adverse side effects with this drug—such as

MAHARISHI REJUVENATION THERAPY

Physiological and Psychological Improvements Through Maharishi Vedic Medicine

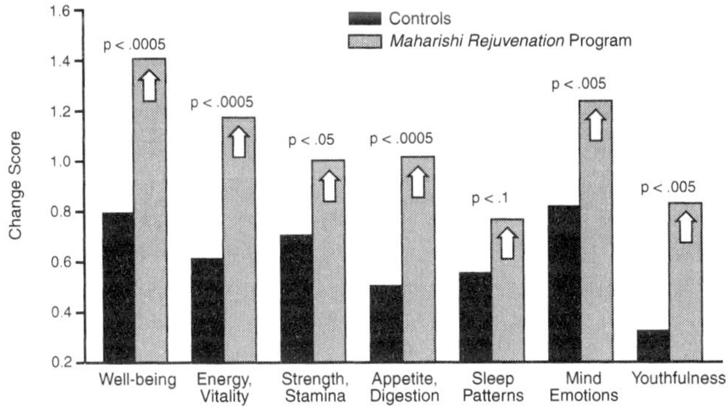

This study found that people who participated in a one-week Maharishi Rejuvenation℠ program of the Maharishi Vedic Approach to Health improved significantly across a wide range of measures. Control subjects who received only intellectual knowledge of this program and its principles for the same amount of time did not show the same amount of improvement. These findings indicate that the Maharishi Rejuvenation program, which is recommended to be applied seasonally to remove accumulated physiological toxins of the season, promotes physiological and psychological balance.

Another study, published in a German medical journal, examined various physiological and psychological changes that occurred in subjects participating in a two-week Maharishi Rejuvenation program. Improvements included reduced cholesterol and urea, reduced bodily complaints and strains, reduced irritability and psychological inhibition, and greater stability and openness.

References: 1. R.H. Schneider, K.L. Cavanaugh, H.S. Kasture, S. Rothenberg, R. Averbach, D. Robinson, And R.K. Wallace, "Health Promotion with a Traditional System of Natural Health Care: Maharishi Ayur-Veda," *Journal of Social Behavior and Personality*, 5 (3) (1990), pp. 1-27

2. R. Waldschutz, "Influence of Maharishi Ayur-Veda Purification Treatment on Physiological and Psychological Health," *Erfahrungsheilkunde-Acta Medica Empirica*, 11 (1988), pp. 720-729.

uterine bleeding, swollen or tender breasts, bloating, nausea, and mood swings, to name a few. It may be good for short-term relief of menopause symptoms, or those at risk for osteoporosis, but long-term effects are still not completely known.

At age 57 Beth Ann came to me with a host of complaints. She was taking HRT for hot flashes but felt uncomfortable with it. Before her hot flashes started, she had tried a number of vitamins and mineral supplements to help with her digestive problems, but they didn't help with the hot flashes. She also had allergies for which she was taking allergy shots. She wanted to get off HRT and try natural herbs.

This is a common desire among menopausal women. Statistics show that only 30 percent of women who are given prescriptions for hormone replacement therapy ever fill them. Of those who fill their prescriptions, more than half of them stop taking the pills within a year.[9] For one thing, women just don't want to take them, and for another, there is great confusion on the subject even within the medical community. New studies seem to come along daily on the benefits and side effects of HRT.

This is the big difference between Western medicine and Maharishi Vedic Medicine. Western medicine can be very useful in the short term, if your life is in a crisis. But menopause is not a crisis situation, it is a natural process in a woman's evolution and should be thought of as such. The ancient texts have long recognized the value of rejuvenating herbs at this stage of life to prevent or alleviate menopausal symptoms. Rather than being a synthetic formula with unknown results, Ayurvedic herbs have long provided women with natural food precursors of estrogen and progesterone.

Some women undergoing menopause have a difficult time and HRT may be required while the mind and body imbalances are being addressed with a comprehensive Ayurvedic program. I don't mean to imply that having a difficult time should be expected with menopause. Having a difficult time during menopause is not the standard experience. For most women, a regular Ayurvedic program prescribed by a physician trained in Maharishi Ayur-Veda which addresses their imbalances will be enough.

For most women experiencing natural menopause, the decision

to seek prescription treatment will be based on four factors:

- the severity of their short-term complaints
- their attitudes toward both menopause and medication
- their predispositions to developing heart disease or osteoporosis
- the potential risks and benefits of each available treatment

Every woman can and should make positive changes in her daily life that will reduce her risk of heart disease, osteoporosis and other age-related diseases, while at the same time increase her good health in all areas in a natural way. While taking estrogen does reduce cholesterol and the risk of heart disease, so do such natural factors as a healthy diet, moderate exercise, and the practice of the TM technique, Maharishi Vedic Medicine and rasayanas—without side effects, by promoting the body's healing mechanisms.

A physician trained in Maharishi Ayur-Veda will look at you as an individual and your lifestyle to determine the Vata/Pitta/Kapha balance, which will be a better tool for recommending a complete program for long-term comfort and a healthy post-menopause life.

Maharishi Vedic Medicine understands that each woman's hormone level is unique to her physiology and varies daily. A synthetic hormone comes into your body in fixed amounts and at a fixed rate, whereas when your biological intelligence regulates the dosage, the amount and rate will vary in subtle and precise ways at different times of the day and under varying conditions. Therefore, many women undergoing HRT are receiving inappropriate amounts of hormones, to a greater or lesser degree.[10]

Breast Cancer

Dana was diagnosed with breast cancer and had 6 1/2 weeks of radiation therapy before seeing me. She also had had a complete hysterectomy. She came to me with concerns of having no natural hormones, and she was concerned about long-term problems with heart disease and osteoporosis. Her current symptoms were persistent hot flashes, chronic migraines, sleeplessness, mood swings, a lot of anger and depression. In addition, she had acne and a skin rash.

Dana felt she was an intelligent and informed consumer and she sought Maharishi Vedic Medicine after reading my book *Forever Healthy*[11] because she said she wanted a more comprehensive and holistic approach to treating the root cause of her problems rather than just the symptoms. She had tried other types of alternative therapies but with minimal relief.

Although breast cancer is not as related to menopause as are heart disease and osteoporosis, it is related to the choice of taking hormone replacement therapy. Many women who come to see me with menopausal concerns ask about breast cancer. A study showed that for a medical practice that includes 2,000 healthy women over the age of 50, every year 20 women will develop heart disease, 11 will develop osteoporosis, six will develop breast cancer, and three will develop endometrial cancer.[12]

Please understand that statistics can be very misleading. Although women have a one in eight chance of developing breast cancer, that risk is for a lifetime. "You have to live to be 90 before you become a one in eight person. The statistics are confusing, and they upset women," states Marilyn Rhodes, RN, BSN, OCN, oncology resource nurse at the City of Hope National Medical Center.

Most women are probably aware that taking any chemical or "natural" hormone can have many unknown effects on the body. Some of these effects are known and some are not. The third major report of the *Nurses' Health Study* documented a 43 percent increase in death from breast cancer in long-term users of hormone replacement therapy.[13] Another study funded by the Imperial Cancer Research Fund, a United Kingdom charity, found that the increase in breast cancer in current and recent users of a combination of estrogen and progestin was greatest in women with lower body weight.[14]

Breast cancer is very much related to our fatty, toxic Western diet. Experts agree that environmental factors, such as diet, account for 80 percent of breast cancers, and genetic factors account for 20 percent. They point the finger at diets high in animal fats and refined carbohydrates. Fats can also contain fat-soluble toxins and xenoestrogens, which either increase cell stress or promote cancer-causing changes.[15]

Pesticides and herbicides in our food are also a concern. According to Robert Herron, Ph.D., a research scientist at the Institute of Science, Technology and Public Policy at Maharishi University of Management in Fairfield, Iowa, "Toxins such as DDT, DDE and DDD are difficult to get out of the physiology, because when they get into the body they have an affinity for fat tissue and embed themselves in it. Even vegetarians who eat a low-fat diet, but one that isn't organic and therefore is loaded with toxic chemicals, are susceptible to the development of breast cancer."[16]

More pesticides are used on fruits and vegetables than on the grain used as feed for animals. Therefore, people who eat only nonorganic fruits and vegetables have a higher potential of exposure to toxic chemicals. Also, toxins from chemicals are in processed dairy products like cheese, yogurt, butter and milk. Because the breasts are primarily made of fat, and toxins are fat soluble, the breasts become a primary storage area for environmental chemicals.

Toxins enter into the physiology primarily through the process of food and water consumption. Food and water contaminated with these compounds enter through the digestive system; or airborne toxins are inhaled and then passed through the lungs into the body. Environmental chemicals (in our food, water, soil and air) harm the DNA cells, the root cells of the physiology. Some can cause cancer over time. Levels of these chemicals in fatty tissues may either remain relatively constant over time or increase with continued exposure. They leave the body primarily in urine, but also in breast milk. Many scientists believe that they are the primary reason for the development of breast cancer.

It is interesting to note that the public knows little of how many pesticides and herbicides are in their food. Even though DDT has been banned in the U.S., it still reaches our produce counters from imported foods. A March 1999 *Consumer Reports* warned parents not to feed their children too many peaches, apples, pears and spinach because of potential pesticide residue. The study recommended buying organically grown produce which has little or no residue.

In Dana's case, I recommended immediate changes in her diet—eating organic foods whenever possible. I also recommended specific Maharishi Vedic Medicine herbal prescriptions, Maharishi Yoga asanas, breathing techniques, oil self-massage and most importantly the practice of the TM technique.

After one month she told me, "I feel pretty good, especially considering my medical problems have been with me for the last few years and more disabling for the last six months. The diet has made a very big change for me. Although I do miss eating oranges and grapefruit (a specific recommendation I made in her case), I have fewer headaches and I'm sleeping better, though not continuously. I have more energy." The following month her depression and anxiety decreased. She was experiencing less anger, and a lower back pain that had followed her hysterectomy surgery had improved dramatically. Her skin rash also cleared up.

Dana felt the most difficult thing to do was the warm oil self-massage because she didn't like using oil. "But I do feel good afterwards," she said. She did learn the TM technique and said that she experienced much more balance and hope for resolution with her chronic disease. I explained to her that the purpose of the TM technique is really to bring a balance in the nervous system, whereby all the other systems in the physiology are consequently balanced. The periods of illness get shorter and the periods of wellness becomes prolonged until someday all the disease can be eliminated. I told her that in the silence of the transcendental field of life all healing and rejuvenation takes place, and in that self-referral state, perfection in the physiology becomes a reality. Dana understood that and continues with all the healing aspects of Maharishi Vedic Medicine.

When Ruth, a 49-year-old systems analyst, came to see me she was already in menopause. Two years previously she had breast cancer and had a lumpectomy with auxiliary lymph nodes removed. She was then put on the drug Tamoxifen. Now she was worried about osteoporosis and the possibility of breast cancer recurrence.

As with other women who come to see me at this time of their lives, she had other problems that she related to menopause. She had difficulty sleeping; continuous lower back pain; chronic indigestion with gas, bloating and reflux (a flowing back, as the food returns to the esophagus from the stomach). She was prone to constipation, which is very common when the gut becomes too dry due to a Vata imbalance. She also noticed that she had dry skin.

Along with dietary changes, I recommended she take the special herbal preparation Maharishi Amrit Kalash on a regular basis to strengthen her immune system. I also recommended Maharishi rejuvenation and purification treatments at a Maharishi Ayur-Veda Health Center to help her physiology eliminate the harmful side effects she was experiencing from her breast cancer treatments. Preliminary studies on the positive effects of these purification treatments show that they are one of the few efficient ways to rid the body of the build-up of harmful toxins. To help relieve the anxiety and fear of recurring cancer, I also encouraged her to learn the TM technique.

Having learned the TM technique, she felt more secure with her treatment. She told me that she understood that the whole purpose of Maharishi Vedic Medicine is to really rejuvenate, bring back balance in the physiology, and to improve immunity. All the approaches of Maharishi Vedic Medicine: diet, exercise, herbal preparations, the TM technique, etc., work towards this goal. Even by incorporating a few of the suggestions from this new health routine, one can benefit enormously. I also told her that strength comes from within—the strength to deal with the fears and worries without skepticism—all that comes from within. When a woman develops that self-referral state, the silent state at the core of the physiology, through regular practice of the TM technique, she can develop the strength, endurance, peace and joy that is needed to overcome the shadows that are created by the fear of cancer.

Later she said to me, "Overall I feel well. I have less back pain and dryness now, and the reflux is better." Later she told me she was sleeping much better and for the most part her reflux had completely disappeared. After her rejuvenation and purification treatments, she had a routine thyroid function test that indicated that she needed to use much less medication. Subsequently her thyroid medication was reduced to half of the dosage she had been taking.

Fibrocystic Breast Disease

Tender, sensitive and swollen breasts can be a problem in menopause due to the development of fibrocystic tissue. This is a Kapha disorder. Paying special attention to massaging the breast area during your recommended warm oil self-massage (see the chapter on daily routine) will improve the circulation of the mastic tissue and encourage lymphatic drainage. A Kapha-reducing diet may be recommended at this time. As a reminder of this diet, avoid dairy products, cold food and drinks, meats, wheat and all sweets except honey. Remember to do your Maharishi Yoga asanas.

Your physician trained in Maharishi Ayur-Veda can give you specific prescriptions for this disease. In my own practice I have had some patients who were able to totally eliminate this disease.

Weighing Benefits Versus Risks

Many short-term menopausal disturbances, and even risk of serious disease later on in life, can be reduced by stopping smoking, as well as exercising and eating right. With proper balance in your lifestyle, most if not all menopause-related disturbances decrease or disappear. During the menopause transition there are ample benefits from learning to manage your own lifestyle in the way that makes sense to you. Knowing that the upsets of menopause are temporary, and that you can choose to look at the remainder of your life as a time of stability and serenity, will bring joy and happiness at this time.

References

1. Lee, J.R. 1996. *What Your Doctor May Not Tell You About Menopause.* New York: Warner Books, p. 35.
2. Lennon, H.M., Wotiz, H.H., Parsons, L., & Mozden, P.J. 1966. Reduced estriol excretion in patients with breast cancer prior to endocrine therapy. *JAMA* 196,112–20.
3. *What Your Doctor May Not Tell You About Menopause,* p. 37.
4. Glaser, J.L., Brind, J.L., Vogelman, J.H. et al. 1992. Elevated serum DHEA-S levels in practitioners of the Transcendental Meditation and TM-Sidhi programs. *Journal of Behavioral Medicine,* 15(4), 327–341.
5. *What Your Doctor May Not Tell You About Menopause,* p. 36.
6. Ellison, P.T., Panter-Brick, C. Lipson, S.F., & O'Rourke, M.T. 1993. The ecological context of human ovarian function. *Human Reproduction,* 8, 2248–58.
7. *What Your Doctor May Not Tell You About Menopause,* p. 47.
8. Grodstein, F., Stampfer, M.J., Colditz, G.A., et al.1997 Postmenopausal Hormone Therapy and Mortality. *New England Journal of Medicine,* 336, 1769–1775.
9. Love, S.M., & Lindsey, K. 1997. *Dr. Susan Love's Hormone Book.* New York: Random House, Introduction, p. xvi.
10. Lonsdorf, N., Butler, V., & Brown, M. 1993. *A Woman's Best Medicine: Health Happiness and Long Life Through Ayur-Veda.*

Tarcher/Putnam, New York, p. 277.

11. Reddy, K. *Forever Healthy.* Schenectady, NY: Samhita Productions.
12. Grady, D., Rubin, S.M, Petitti, D.B. et al. 1992. Hormone therapy to prevent disease and prolong life in postmenopausal women. *Ann Intern Med,* 117, 1017.
13. Grodstein, F., Stampfer, M.J., Colditz, G.A., et al.1997. Postmenopausal hormone therapy and mortality. *New England Journal of Medicine,* 336, 1769–1775.
14. Collaborative Group on Hormonal Factors in Breast Cancer. 1997. *Lancet,* 350, 1047–1059.
15. *What Your Doctor May Not Tell You About Menopause,* pp. 211–213.
16. Herron, R. 1999. *Removing Environmental Toxins with Maharishi Rejuvenation and Purification.* A videotaped speech. The Raj Maharishi Ayur-Veda Health Center, Fairfield, IA.

CHAPTER ELEVEN

Other Problems Associated with Menopause

Almost every woman who comes into my office with menopausal concerns mentions that she wants to lose weight. Often women associate personal power with how they look, and at this time they really want to look and feel their best. A survey by *American Health Magazine* indicated that men are more interested in sex when they feel fit and in shape, while women feel sexier when they weigh less. Weight, then, for women, seems to be more of a concern of appearance than health.

Weight Gain

When Jean came to see me she was perimenopausal and experiencing a lot of marital stress. Her average weight had been 125 pounds but she currently weighed 185 pounds. She had been taking a drug for depression for the last several years and she was experiencing migraine headaches, PMS, weeping spells, moodiness and anxiety. Jean felt she was not her usual self and that her "sharp tongue" wasn't helping her marriage problems. She couldn't seem to lose any weight, although she had tried all kinds of diet regimens.

A woman's metabolism changes during and after menopause. Everyone's metabolism begins to slow during the early to mid-30s. The number of calories needed by women declines between 2 and 8 percent for every decade after their twentieth birthday.[1] This change occurs slowly, so it may take a while for the impact of poor eating habits to affect weight. Unfortunately, the change from pre- to post-menopausal status is associated with increased waist circumference, decreased hip circumference, and increased waist-to-hip ratio.[2] Diets high in animal fats, sugar, refined starches, and processed foods lead to estrogen levels in women living in industrially advanced countries that are twice as high as those in third-world countries. This leads to exaggerated estrogen decline at menopause.[3]

Let's not even get into what a "normal" weight should be. Different people have fat distributed in different areas. What is considered obese in some cultures is considered a beauty advantage in another. Thin and young do not necessarily equate.

However, if you feel sluggish, have too many rolls of fat, tire easily, don't exercise, and experience unhappiness whenever you look at yourself in the mirror, chances are you need to take off excess fat.

For women especially, being even slightly overweight is a distressing and embarrassing condition. It is associated with a number of medical complications, many of which are life-threatening. Each year, Americans spend approximately $100 million on obesity-related health and diet food products.[4]

By now you realize that it is a factor of imbalance in a predominantly Kapha physiology. Both Western medicine and Maharishi Vedic Medicine agree on this: exercise is the key to creating and maintaining a balanced physiology. This is especially true for the Kapha woman. Thin is not a key-word here—balance and well-being are what is sought. Often, the laid-back Kapha type *hates* to exercise. What to do?

In Maharishi Vedic Medicine there is a phrase which says, "what you put your attention on grows." For those who need to lose weight, the attention should go to positive addictions such as exercise, especially Maharishi Yoga asanas, the Transcendental Meditation technique, which helps reduce stress (and therefore, helps reduce overeating due to stress). And eat fresh, organic foods which are acceptable for your physiology at the proper time of day. Eating balanced meals with all six tastes is of primary importance. By pacifying Kapha and creating a strong agni (digestive fire), balance can be restored in the physiology and the weight will come off.

This is the time of your life when you need to look after yourself, pay attention to your body's needs, stop feeding yourself emotionally, take means to eliminate stress from your life and, basically, be a mature, healthy woman of wisdom.

When Jean started to diet, she caused Pitta to swing out of balance because she wasn't feeding herself enough. This caused her to be "sharp-tongued." Skipping meals can also create ama in the physiology and cause sluggishness. Constant dieting had thrown Jean's digestion out of kilter. Ayurvedic texts state that digestion, assimilation and metabolism are vital not only for overall health, but for energy, clarity of mind and lustrous skin.

I advised Jean to eat her main meal at midday when digestion is the strongest, and to eat a lighter meal at night. I also told her not to eat leftovers or cold foods—she was incorrectly eating salads, which were not good for her. Fresh, organic, cooked foods, no heavy foods or dairy products at night, and no hurried meals were part of Jean's new dietary regimen. To help balance her cravings and appetite, I had her take an Ayurvedic digestive aid and use the Maharishi Ayur-Veda seasonings called *churnas* to help her to get all six tastes at her meals. A spicy type of tea was recommended to help her with cravings. Jean was also not getting enough exercise nor was she taking time for herself. I recommended both.

As Jean started to incorporate the routines suggested by Maharishi Vedic Medicine's approach to health, she started feeling much better. Her digestion and all areas of her physiology improved. She lost weight and reduced her depression medication. In two months her weight came down to 150 pounds and she found that her PMS symptoms had diminished. She started sleeping better and had more energy.

Jean said, "My mental and emotional PMS are under control. I feel mentally and spiritually great!" Five months later she wanted to eliminate her drug medication completely. I advised her to do it slowly.

Skin Problems

At menopause, when a woman enters the Vata Kala time of her life, skin changes can occur. These changes usually show up on the face. Because dryness is associated with Vata, even if you've only had few skin problems before, some drying can occur which, if not corrected, can cause unwanted lines on the face. Excess Pitta can cause acne, especially around the nose and chin area. Excess Kapha produces too much oil that can lead to clogged pores. Actually, any imbalance in the physiology can appear on the face as aging.

Hormonal changes can cause numerous skin problems. Since estrogen is necessary for smooth, hydrated skin, when levels are low or in flux, the consequent increase in sebaceous secretions often produces acne in sensitive and oily skin. Stress, in general, can cause the skin to become dehydrated and the pH levels to change. Worry lines can appear. An unhealthy diet consisting of excess coffee and caffeine, carbonated sodas, and too many sweets can cause damage. Dwelling on negativity can put lines on your face, too.

Another problem can be due to too much Pitta where the agni is too high. Skin rashes, hot flashes, and the heating of the body in general are all signs that Pitta dosha wants attention. Spicy, sour, fermented (soy sauces, vinegar) foods should be avoided. Also, the hot spices like cayenne and pepper should be avoided.

Spritzing your face with refreshing rose water is not only good for the skin, but immediately calms Pitta. Rose water can be used for all the doshas to help protect and give elasticity and firmness to the skin. Speaking of elasticity, Maharishi Yoga asanas—particularly the ones that send blood to the face—are an excellent way of reversing the aging process on the face, and, in fact, the whole body. You can learn these asanas at a Maharishi Ayur-Veda Health Center.

A weak agni can give you a dull complexion, because toxins and excess wastes are not being removed properly from your system and they can cause a dullness to your complexion. Poor circulation, often a Kapha imbalance, will also make the skin dull.

Ojas is the end product of a good digestion and a healthy diet. It is the subtle substance that gives healthy skin its natural glow. When ojas is low, the immune response is weak and the skin becomes lifeless. A strong immune system and beautiful skin require strong ojas, a balanced constitution, and the proper transformation and function of the dhatus and malas.

A warm oil self-massage once a day (sluggish Kaphas can do one twice a day) is probably the best thing you can do topically for your skin. Herbal beauty care is a timeless tradition that, in ancient times, both men and women performed. Maharishi Ayur-Veda has natural skin products that are remarkable in their use of natural ingredients.

To nourish your skin eat a diet full of fresh organic foods, not lifeless processed foods:

- eat lots of fresh, sweet, juicy fruits like pears, plums and ripe melons (if you have a Kapha imbalance, best to follow a Kapha-balancing diet first)
- eat green leafy vegetables and carrots
- avoid carbonated beverages
- avoid ice cold drinks
- drink plenty of water

Special skin programs, which use rose water, special muds, herbs and organic milks, are available at some Maharishi Ayur-Veda Health Centers (See the Index for a list of Maharishi Ayur-Veda Health Centers.)

Sleep Disorders

The quality of your sleep is so very important. According to the

Charaka Samhita, sleep is one of the main supports of your physiology. If you have good quality sleep, you will wake up happy.

Because an out-of-balance Vata-type woman can be mentally irritated and have anxiety, she often has trouble falling asleep. An increase in Vata dosha, which happens naturally at menopause, can create an unsettled, worrisome mind or nervous system. Insomnia is also related to other Vata imbalances, such as constipation caused by Vata's drying qualities, fatigue, or restlessness (due to Vata moving in the physiology). Often women say they are too tired to sleep. That is a sign of Vata moving in the physiology.

In my practice I always give a comprehensive approach of proper diet, exercise and herbal prescriptions. In addition to this, I often recommend herbal tablets, special herb tea, and aroma oil to help calm Vata dosha. Simple lavender oil helps relax the physiology as well. Special herbal tablets help calm all the doshas. These over-the-counter preparations can be obtained from a Maharishi Ayur-Veda products catalog. These herbals can be used in addition to a comprehensive program given to you by physicians trained in Maharishi Ayur-Veda.

Another way of keeping Vata dosha calm is a soothing warm sesame oil foot massage to the soles of your feet before going to bed. Going to bed before 10 p.m. will help settle Vata. Also, don't watch TV or read before going to bed, or eat dry foods such as crackers. Deep breathing also helps relax Vata.

Waking up during the night full of energy is a symptom of an imbalance in Pitta dosha. Hot flashes during the night will create sleep problems and is a common complaint at menopause. Balancing Pitta dosha can help with both problems. Pitta can become aggravated when meals are skipped, or are too spicy, which can cause Pitta anger to flare up. Eating sweet, juicy fruits and taking Rose Petal Conserve in 1/2 cup of cool milk or soy milk can help calm Pitta.

If you are skipping meals in order to lose weight, don't. Skipping meals creates ama. Eat a light meal, soup or light grains and vegetables, at least two hours before retiring.

Besides balancing Vata and Pitta doshas, Maharishi Ayur-Veda often recommends drinking a cup of organic, boiled, warm milk at night right before going to bed. This soothes the physiology. A pinch of nutmeg and/or cardamom can be added. Sometimes a small teaspoon of liquefied ghee is added to help with dry bowels.

A sign of Kapha imbalance is too much sleep, feeling drowsy during the day, and not feeling truly rested. Ama is clogging the channels that signal the body to sleep more. This can create unhappiness and depression. A warm oil self-massage in the evening can help a sluggish physiology. Exercise, of course, but not right before bedtime. Over exercise can cause sleeplessness. Dietary corrections are most important for Kapha types. A short, healthful fast may put Kapha back in line. Avoid lots of sweet, cold, heavy foods. Eat more spicy foods or a small slice of fresh ginger before meals. Use cumin, coriander and turmeric in your food. Sip warm water, or warm water with ginger added.

Headaches

Headaches can be caused by the emotions or by many other factors including allergies, caffeine withdrawal, digestive problems, tension, working too long in front of a computer, or focusing too much on negativity.

Carolyn, an artist, was suffering from migraine headaches. In addition to her busy schedule she was also taking care of an elderly parent. At age 57, she was post-menopause. She had a history of high blood pressure which had started at age 35 and she had been on medication since then.

When Carolyn came to see me she was taking Hytrin for her high blood pressure, which was making her agitated at night so she was unable to sleep. Carolyn also had frequent urination, chronic indigestion, hot flashes, muscle cramps in her toes, and arthritis in her neck. She was receiving treatments for arthritis and her migraines, but she wasn't having much relief.

A person's constitution determines the remedy. Maharishi Vedic Medicine sees an imbalance of Vata dosha as leading to stiffness or constipation, the strain of which can cause a throbbing sensation in the head. A Vata-pacifying diet can help with constipation and insomnia. Massaging tension spots in the body, especially in the neck and shoulders with warm sesame oil followed by a warm shower helps pacify Vata. A light massage on the soles of the feet before going to bed will sooth Vata. Drinking plenty of fresh warm water throughout the day can be very helpful. Dehydration can cause headaches. Sometimes a headache can be eliminated by drinking a glass or two of water.

Pitta can become aggravated by too spicy or hot food, which can create a headache. Or, as the eyes tend to overwork, strain in the eye area can cause a headache just behind the eyes. Bright light, hot sun, excessive heat can all aggravate Pitta. Wearing a head covering and cool clothing can help prevent headaches.

Sometimes eating something sweet, like a sweet, juicy fruit, will sooth Pitta. If someone with a predominance of Pitta suddenly stops drinking caffeinated soft drinks, coffee or tea, a headache can occur. A sip or two of a caffeinated beverage will stop the headache, if that is the cause. To prevent future headaches, cut out caffeine slowly. Pitta types should be careful to not hold in anger or tenseness. Soothing aromatherapy oils diffused while sleeping can help restore balance and prevent headaches.

Kapha types can get sinus headaches or headaches due to hay fever or allergies. Burning a stimulating Kapha aroma oil which contains eucalyptus will help with mild congestion. Certain Maharishi Yoga asanas can also help with headaches.

Carolyn's immediate response to her treatment of learning the Transcendental Meditation technique to reduce her high blood pressure, dietary and herbal recommendations, aromatherapy, massage therapy, and detoxification programs, was that her digestion improved dramatically, her energy level went up, her muscle cramps and joint pain lessened. Whereas she wasn't walking before, she started walking for exercise. She could do this now because her joint pain was better.

She said, "I got better despite being irregular in taking my herbs. I forget to take them sometimes. I am also very irregular with my oil

INNER HAPPINESS

Increased Self-Actualization Through the *Transcendental Meditation* Technique

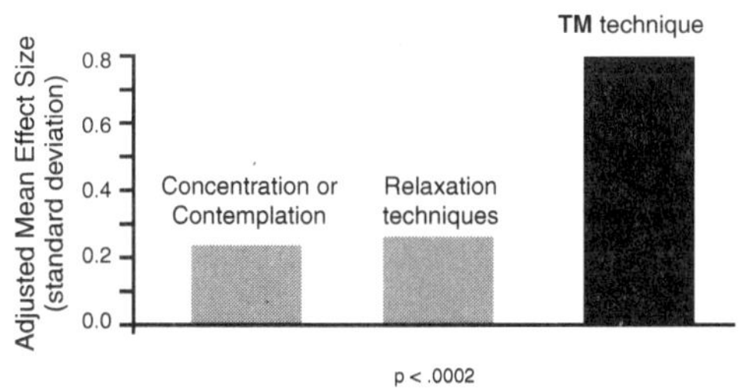

Statistical meta-analysis of all available studies (42 independent outcomes) indicated that the effect of the Transcendental Meditation program on increasing self-actualization is much greater then concentration, contemplation, or relaxation techniques. Self-actualization refers to realizing more of one's inner potential, expressed in every area of life: integration and stability of personality, self-regard, emotional maturity, capacity for warm interpersonal relationships, and adaptive response to challenges.

Reference: C.N. Alexander, M. Rainforth and P. Gelderloos, "TM, Self-Actualization, and Psychological Health: A Conceptual Overview and Statistical Meta-Analysis," *Journal of Social Behavior and Personality*, 6 (1991), pp. 189-247.

Orientation Towards Positive Values

In three studies of college students, practitioners of the Transcendental Meditation and TM-Sidhi programs exhibited more positive attitudes and perceptions than did controls, in terms of memory, recognition threshhold, and interpersonal appraisal.

Reference: P. Gelderloos, P.H. Goddard III, H.H.B. Ahlstrom, and R. Jacoby, "Cognitive Orientation Toward Positive Values in Advanced Participants of the TM and TM-Sidhi Program," *Perceptual and Motor Skills*, 64 (1987) pp. 1003-1012.

massage. But I feel much better when I follow the program and I feel more tired when I don't." Her blood pressure came back to normal in less than three months, so she decided to stop the blood pressure medication that she had been taking for years.

Carolyn's neck pain dramatically improved. She learned to take better care of her neck once she understood that cold weather or very humid weather could aggravate the discomfort. At the end of seven months she said, "I have less pain. This is the first winter I have experienced less pain. I'm really impressed. I am more than impressed that my blood pressure has been very good despite my stressful job and living environment." Her muscle cramps and headaches—mostly a sign of Vata aggravation—have completely gone.

Genitourinary Problems

Common problems in this age group include urinary frequency, frequent urinary tract infections, and urinary incontinence. They need to be evaluated carefully. Urinary frequency can be seen in a variety of conditions like diabetes; excessive intake of water, caffeine and soft drinks; diseases of the bladder, kidney and liver, and even the heart. It can also be due to prescription medications. I have seen many women who responded very well with dietary changes and Maharishi Vedic Medicine herbs, and they did not need HRT.

Frequent urinary tract infections indicate lowered immunity. Other pathological reasons like stones and tumors need to be ruled out. In my practice many women get good relief with Maharishi Vedic Medicine treatments without the need for HRT or antibiotics. Long-term use of antibiotics have many undesirable side effects.

Urinary incontinence is considered a Vata imbalance. It can be due to poor muscle tone of the pelvic floor muscles, estrogen deficiency, and aging. Yoga asanas which strengthen pelvic floor muscles are recommended. There are specific herbal preparations to help this problem in its early stages.

Some women experience lower sexual desire, vaginal dryness, painful intercourse, etc. Remember Jean who came in to see me for hot flashes, weight gain, loss of libido and occipital neuralgia. In less than three months all her symptoms were gone including the loss of libido. Dietary changes, specific herbs, yoga asanas and massage helped her. Treatment is customized to the individual woman. Every woman is unique and special and needs specialized treatment.

References

1. Jacobowitz, R.S. 1993. *150 Most-Asked Questions About Menopause.* New York: William Morrow and Company, p. 200.
2. Caterson, I.D. 1990. Management strategies for weight control, eating, exercise, and behavior. *Drugs,* 39 (supplement 3), 20.
3. Lee, J.R.1996. *What Your Doctor May Not Tell You About Menopause.* New York: Warner Books, p. 40.
4. Atkinson, R.L. 1993. Proposed standards for judging the success of the treatment of obesity. *Ann Intern Med,* 1(19), 677.

CHAPTER TWELVE

Dealing with Emotions

Alberta was only 42 when she started having irregular and delayed periods, which signaled the onset of perimenopause. When she did have a period, it was a heavy flow accompanied with pain. She also had been suffering with irritable bowel syndrome for several years. Chronic indigestion, heartburn, anxiety with disturbed sleep were also on Alberta's list of problems. She had been an alcoholic. However, by the time she came to see me, she had been sober for four years.

Her major life-negating habit was smoking. Smoking is not only hazardous to the lungs, but is a major contributing factor to heart disease as well as osteoporosis. Alberta had been smoking two packs of cigarettes per day since her teens. She had started smoking to deal with the stress caused by "a broken heart" as a teenager and just never stopped. It was a habit she wanted to break but her body and mind were very addicted. Smoking is not a stress-reduction technique. It is a life-negating technique.

When Alberta came to see me she was wise enough in the ways of the world to understand that she no longer needed smoking as an emotional crutch, but she was having a hard time stopping. She had also looked into her family's health history and she was worried, rightfully, about the effects her bad habits were having on her heart. Intense emotional stress was coming to play in Alberta's life at this time—a frequent occurrence in women when they begin perimenopause.

Your Heart, Head and Emotions Are Connected

Your brain and your heart are intricately connected, and because of this, your thoughts and emotions have a powerful effect on the heart's rhythm. Sudden cardiac death, which is caused by a fatal arrhythmia known as ventricular fibrillation is an electrical instability of the heart muscle, which results in a failure of the heart to pump blood. It is considered the number one medical disorder in the world. This sudden cardiac death is not associated with diet or exercise but with "psycho-social" stress. This makes *stress* the number one medical disorder in the world in both industrial and agrarian societies. "Stress kills" is a reality.

Coronary disease does not develop overnight, and it often manifests at the time of menopause, because estrogen's protective effect can be minimal at that time. As Dr. Christiane Northrup puts it, "A considerable number of women—even healthy women—experience heart palpitations around the time of menopause. These palpitations generally do NOT indicate heart disease. There's no question that heart palpitations at menopause are related to changing hormones."[1] But both results, coronary disease and problems with changes occurring at menopause, are due to poor choices in lifestyle—especially in the area of stress release.

Because your thoughts and emotions have a powerful effect on the heart's rhythm, how you interpret events that happen to you can cause your own heart to "break" or be damaged in some way emotionally. Negative emotions like anger, hate, or fear release a rush of neurochemicals that strain and damage the organs. Worry (a Vata disorder) especially weakens the heart. Positive emotions like love and laughter release health-promoting chemicals. This again is where practicing the Transcendental Meditation technique and participating in Maharishi Ayur-Veda rejuvenation therapies can help you unlock old emotions and get through and over stresses, thus helping restore your physiology to its proper inner wisdom.

As Dr. Northrup says—"Think of it (psycho-social stress) this way: the emotional and psychological changes that take place during perimenopause affect your entire life cycle the same way that the week before your period affects your monthly cycle. In other words, all of the issues that have been coming up premenstrually (should I quit my job, should I stay in this relationship) come back and hit you at mid-life."[2]

Many bad habits have an effect on the heart—improper diet, lack of exercise, negative thoughts (which create ama in the physiology). Heart attacks do not happen by coincidence to those who are very overweight or under exercised. In a Johns Hopkins' study, Dr. Jerilyn Allen, RN, ScD., stated that "Women who gain 5 to 8 kilograms (11 to 17.6 pounds) are 25 percent more likely to develop coronary disease. . . . That's not a real big weight gain; it's common."[3]

In Western medicine, a wide range of drugs are available to treat the various forms of heart disease which is the result of poor lifestyle. The thinking runs along these lines: eliminate the pathogen responsible for a symptom and this will restore health. Unfortunately, even if the drug helps with the condition, the disease itself is likely to recur. If a patient with coronary artery disease, characterized by inadequate blood flow through clogged arteries, does not improve with various drugs, surgery may be performed. Most women don't want to go that route. These methods are designed to combat the end point or symptoms of the disease and not the causal factors of lifestyle or environment.

Upon my recommendation Alberta immediately learned the Transcendental Meditation technique and started a comprehensive Maharishi Vedic Medicine program. As you recall Maharishi Vedic Medicine focuses on the origin of the symptoms, rather than the symptoms themselves. It recommends Maharishi Yoga asana stretches (which every body type can perform), dietary corrections and attention to daily routine. The primary recommendation, however, is the Transcendental Meditation technique. It is the most widely researched and proven method of stress release in the world.

After only two months Alberta told me, "I feel much better. I have had two normal periods and I feel less bloated. I am much calmer with only occasional anxiety, but I am practicing my TM technique regularly. My stomach seems to have settled down. I have difficulty finding time to do my self massage, but I am trying. The big news is that I have only been smoking five to six cigarettes a day (as opposed to two packs)."

A month later Alberta reported that her periods were normal, not heavy. "I continue to get better and I haven't felt this well in a very long time. I still have occasional times of anxiety. I particularly noticed a difference when I went home for the holidays. I didn't meditate or eat regularly. This has convinced me how important it is to follow the recommendations. I feel so much better when I stick to my new routine."

Alberta continues to progress. She has attempted to quit smoking but can't stay off for more than a week. I encouraged her to continue with a small amount of smoking and allow the body to spontaneously quit smoking rather than force it. A lifetime of bad habits cannot be corrected in a day. Fortunately, given the right tools—proper diet, herbal preparations, the TM technique and other life enhancing modifications—the mind and the body will respond much faster than you might think.

The Seat of the Emotions—The Limbic System

Your physiology metabolizes the emotional content of every experience you have. This metabolization happens through the limbic system. The limbic area of the brain that correlates with deep emotional states and is considered to be the physiological seat of emotions. It surrounds the hypothalamus, known as the brain's brain, and is the body's command post. The hypothalamus regulates temperature, thirst, hunger, blood sugar levels, growth, sleeping, waking and the emotions.

The pituitary gland, located below the hypothalamus, emits secretions that control the activity of many other glands in the body.

These three elements—the limbic area, hypothalamus, and pituitary—form the limbic system, which alters with every flux in emotions. This creates a new mix of molecules that transform the functioning of the body.

The hypothalamus receives information from a number of sources—the senses, the immune system, cognitive information and emotion. Stimuli coming from the limbic region of the brain cause the hypothalamus to release a wide variety of neuropeptides. The neuropeptides stimulate specific hormones from the pituitary gland, and therefore, specific activity in all endocrine glands, including the thymus and adrenal glands. This new combination of chemical messengers changes the operation and make-up of the body, especially the metabolic system and the immune system.[4]

Through the action of the limbic system, particular psychological and emotional states take on molecular form. If you have ever seen a movie of flying through the Grand Canyon or flying up and down and around and your stomach lurches even though you are not even moving, this is a sign that chemical messengers have been released. Your physiology has absorbed what you have been watching. Watching a sad movie can make you sad or trigger some other emotion, even though you are not participating in the event. The emotions stirred up by the movie correlate with activity in the limbic system. Your emotions have become metabolized into your physiology.

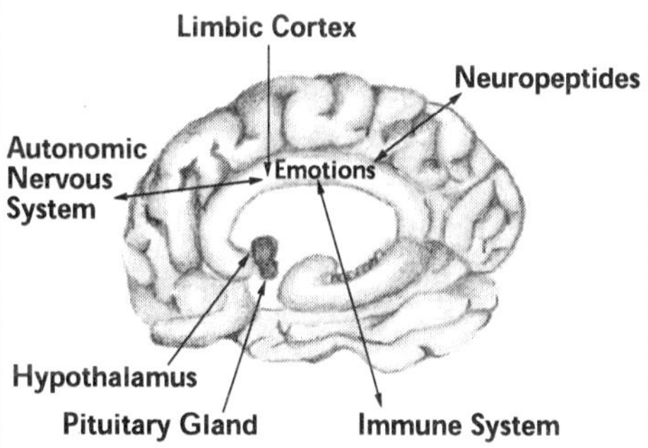

Through the action of the limbic system your physiology metabolizes the emotional content of every expereince you have.

This is another area where the practice of the Transcendental Meditation technique greatly helps. Transcendental

Meditation is said to have an influence through the limbic system. During the practice of this technique, the limbic system metabolizes peace and contentment instead of metabolizing stress.

Lana came to me at age 52 with mood swings, hot flashes and Raynaud's phenomenon, a disease that is thought to be caused by strong emotions or exposure to the cold. In cold weather the fingers, toes, ears or nose become white, due to a lack of blood flow in that area. They then turn blue, which is a result of tiny blood vessels dilating to allow more blood to remain in the tissues. When the flow of blood returns, the area becomes red and then later returns to normal color. There may be associated tingling, swelling, and painful throbbing. The attacks may last anywhere from minutes to hours.

In Lana's case, the Raynaud's disease had started ten years ago. She had also been diagnosed as hypothyroid for the last twenty-two years and she was on replacement therapy. Along with those problems Lana had a skin rash, headaches, lower back pain, and chronic digestive problems since menopause. She was also feeling angry and stressful due to the downsizing of her department. Because of this work stress, she had developed high blood pressure and had gained weight.

I put Lana on a weight loss regimen with herbs that specifically help with weight loss. I made dietary and other recommendations including specific Maharishi Ayur-Veda herbs for menopause, an herbal calcium supplement and aroma therapy. She reported that her hot flashes improved, but due to extreme stress she had developed heart palpitations, and sleep had become erratic. She decided to learn the TM technique. Following this she started to do an oil self-massage in the evenings, which helped her to sleep.

Lana was facing many personal challenges due to her job, but after she began the Maharishi Vedic Medicine program she said she felt "much more calm and less angry." About ten months into her treatment Lana said that she felt balanced and she enjoyed her meditation. She was also experiencing fewer episodes of Raynaud's phenomenon.

Lana continued with the Maharishi Vedic Medicine program and her heart palpitations disappeared completely. She said to me, "I couldn't have handled this whole stress and turmoil if it wasn't for Maharishi Vedic Medicine. I was ready to quit work many times." I advised her to continue with Maharishi Vedic Medicine and to balance her life as much as possible while continuing to work, for she needed the financial resources very much. And, I told her not to confuse life with livelihood.

More about Ojas

Earlier it was stated that ojas is a biochemical substance that has a profound influence on the quality of mental and emotional life. To equate this knowledge in Western medicine, ojas is thought to be equivalent to neuropeptides from the hypothalamus, which have identical effects. Also the ancient texts say that ojas comes from a structure called the *hridaya*. The hridaya is often translated as "heart." Those who translate the Ayurvedic texts suggest that the word heart does not stand for what we know as the circulator pump, but something subtler. One thought is that the hridaya is equivalent to the hypothalamus.[5]

Ayurvedic texts say that happiness is the most effective means of producing ojas. Positive behavior and actions towards others, love, joy and appreciation of life produce ojas, and therefore better immunity.

Other ways to help the body increase ojas is through Ayurvedic purification therapy that removes impurities from the srotas, the physiological channels in the body. This improves the cells' ability to accumulate ojas and rejuvenate the body.

Rasayanas (special Ayurvedic herbal and mineral substances) are defined as "that which causes ojas to be produced all over." (See the chapter on herbs). Special "behavioral rasayanas" also have an effect on health.

Behavioral Rasayanas

In general, the word "rasayana" is used for the substances that strengthen immunity. The term is also used to describe positive ways in which to behave. Western medicine is beginning to understand that the body has its own internal pharmacy that produces substances that influence immune strength. For example, laughter reduces levels of stress hormones such as cortisol and epinephrine, and increases the activity of immune cells such as T cells, natural killer cells and antibodies.[6]

Behavioral rasayanas deal with the mind's influence on the body. They are behaviors that create health-promoting biochemical effects. One result of practicing behavioral rasayanas is that the limbic system is metabolizing positive emotions more often and negative emotions less often.

Behavioral Rasayanas to Be Maximized and to Be Avoided

BEHAVIORS AND ATTITUDES TO BE MAXIMIZED:

- Love
- Compassion
- Speech that uplifts people
- Cleanliness
- Charity and regular donation
- Religious observance
- Respect toward teachers and elders
- Being positive
- Moderation and self-control, especially with regard to alcohol and sex
- Simplicity

TO BE AVOIDED:

- Anger
- Violence
- Harsh or hurtful speech
- Conceit
- Coveting another's spouse or wealth
- Egotism
- Speaking ill of others behind their back
- Dishonesty

The mind is a very strong friend when it comes to handling your emotions wisely. How you interpret the emotional ups and downs experienced at the time of menopause is just as important as taking balancing herbs and purification treatments. And how you

Factors that Diminish Ojas

- Negative emotions of any kind
- Stress
- Hurrying
- Excessive exercise
- Fasting. (Moderate fasting is sometimes used in special doctor-supervised situations in Maharishi Vedic Medicine, but excessive fasting can weaken the body by emaciating the bodily tissues and reducing the ojas which nourishes them.)
- Rough or very light diet
- Overexposure to wind and sun
- Staying awake through most of the night
- Excessive loss of bodily fluids, such as blood
- Overindulgence in sexual activity
- Alcoholic beverages

interpret emotional swings may be strongly influenced by your knowledge of what is going on in your physiology.

Depression

At age 48, Sarah, a hospice health care provider, had been in menopause for a year. She was under stress, emotionally, mentally and physically, which resulted in both anxiety and depression. She had been placed on both anti-anxiety medication and an anti-depressant.

Depression is an emotional state in which there are extreme feelings of sadness, dejection, lack of self worth and emptiness. For recurring episodes of depression, irritability and nervousness, a physician may prescribe antidepressants and tranquilizers or psychotherapy. But these methods do not get at the root cause of depression.

Due to the influence of the advertising media, it is thought that depression is common among perimenopausal and menopausal women. The fact is, menopausal women ages 45 to 64 actually have a lower incidence of depression than younger women.[7] More likely, they are happy that they don't have to bother with having periods anymore.

For most women the time surrounding menopause can be just the same old routine, or fun, or a big upheaval. It may depend on how you interpret aging. Health information on menopause may be biased and reflect negative images of the aging woman. Initial findings from the Massachusetts Women's Health Study, sponsored by the National Institutes of Health, reveal that the majority of women do not seek help concerning natural menopause and their attitudes are overwhelmingly positive or neutral.[8]

Women who are depressed before menopause are likely to be depressed during menopause and perceive menopause as being the cause of their depression. However, studies have failed to support the premise that depression is the result of low estrogen.

If a Vata-type woman becomes depressed, she seems fearful, anxious, nervous and often can't sleep. On the other hand, Pitta can be aggravated by hot foods, temperatures and emotions. A Pitta type will become angry, or be fearful of failure or losing control. She hates to make mistakes and if she is depressed, she will fear that she *is* making mistakes. Her need to be perfect becomes overblown, and she thinks the only way to solve her problem is through quitting all together. She may also become mildly depressed in the winter and be affected by seasonal affective disorder (SAD).

The Kapha-type woman is subject to depression due to her excess weight, which might cause her to sleep too much which just creates more of a problem. Eating heavy, oily foods and feeling lethargic with no energy is often a Kapha-type woman's complaint.

Sarah had more things going on in her physiology than just depression. She had been on estrogen replacement therapy for about six months to help with hot flashes before she came to see me. This had caused her to retain fluids and to increase her frequent headaches, although it did reduce her hot flashes somewhat.

Sarah also thought she had attacks of hypoglycemia and she had gained twenty pounds within one year. She was experiencing tiredness and sleep problems. Because she was tired she would take a nap after work, which caused her not to sleep at night. She had taken homeopathic remedies in the past for short periods of time with marginal relief. Currently she was taking mega vitamins and mineral therapy. She was also on a diet prescribed by a nutritionist.

If clinical depression does arise during this time of change, it is often precipitated by a number of stressful events that have a negative impact on health. Great changes can happen during the menopausal years: children leaving home, divorce, death of a loved one, job changes, moves, any number of things. These changes are *not caused* by menopause and should not be associated with it. Upheavals in your life can be handled more easily through the practice of the Transcendental Meditation technique, corrections in diet, and positive life-style changes.

Sarah was placed on a Maharishi Ayur-Veda diet that was appropriate for balancing her doshas and thereby balancing her weight. She was also recommended to start the Transcendental Meditation technique to help balance her mentally and emotionally. I gave her simple Maharishi Yoga asanas and breathing techniques to help balance the mind and exercise the body. She was put on herbal preparations, which included Maharishi Amrit Kalash, for her various symptoms. And she was encouraged to try different aroma blends, which have an instant balancing effect on the limbic system in the brain.

After Sarah started more balanced eating, exercising regularly, and taking her herbs, her moods became more settled and she started sleeping better—for at least three to four hours at a time, where before she used to wake up every hour. After two weeks she noticed that her headaches were less, her hot flashes had lessened and her hypoglycemic episodes had decreased.

By the end of two months she had eliminated almost all of her symptoms and she was convinced that this program was what she had needed all along. At her two-year follow-up appointment she was relatively symptom-free.

References

1 & 2. Northrup, C., 1999 (May). Heart Palpitations at Menopause: Your Heart's Wake-up Call! *Health Wisdom for Women.*

3. Edelson, M. A. 1999 (June). Woman's heart attack. *Spa Magazine.*

4 & 5. Sharma, H., & Clark, C. 1998. *Contemporary Ayurveda.* Harcourt Brace & Co. p. 32.

6. Hillhouse, J.E., Kiecolt-Glaser, J.K, & Glaser, R. 1991. Stress-associated modulate of the immune response in humans. In Plotnikoff, N.P. et al. *Stress and Immunity,* Boca Raton, FL: CRC, pp. 3-27.

7. Hunter, M.S. 1993. Predictors of menopausal symptoms: Psychological aspects. *Baillieres Clinical Endocrinology and Metabolism,* 7(1), 33–45.

8. Bosarge, P.M., 1998. Menopause: Separating the myths from the truth. *Woman's Health Source Book III,* p. 425.

Chapter Thirteen

Drugs, Vitamins, Herbs, Free Radicals and Rasayanas

Women have concerns about estrogen therapy or any other kind of "chemicals" or synthetic hormones. They have concerns about estrogen therapy because of potential long-term negative effects. They're looking for something else to provide them with symptomatic relief and, with the increased awareness with respect to heart disease and osteoporosis, they're wondering what they can do if they don't want to take estrogen therapy. And because of what happens to women like Becky, who became addicted to the drug she was taking for anti-anxiety and had to go to a rehab center, many women simply will not take drugs.

Today's modern medical school curriculum focuses almost entirely on disease and not prevention through natural means. Perhaps that is why Western medicine has turned menopause into a disease—so that they can "treat" it. Many Western doctors do not know how—because they were not trained—to encourage the body's natural healing mechanisms. When doctors start their medical practices, drug companies send superior sales people to inform them of their latest products and encourage the doctors to use them. The idea of using preparations from plants still seems like an out-of-date idea to many in the medical community even though, not that long ago, most remedies came from plants.

Drugs

Synthetic pharmaceuticals are made to achieve quick, standard and consistent results. If a substance can be manufactured or isolated to do this, then it becomes of use to Western medicine. These drugs have to be separated and isolated from other substances in order to measure them effectively. High-tech medicine is potent, invasive and frequently harmful as evidenced by the amount of drug toxicity caused by modern drugs. The drug invades the body and knocks out the disease, which would be a blessing to everyone except for negative side effects. These negative effects can be anything from itching to death. Or, as happened to Becky, the drugs can become addictive.

According to an article published in the *Journal of the American Medical Association*:[1]

- In 1994 nearly 106,000 hospital patients may have died from adverse drug reactions.
- Approximately 15 percent of all hospital patients experience an adverse drug reaction.

Drugs that produce intense effects very rapidly have their use for the treatment of emergency conditions, where drugs can save a person's life. But for management of most illnesses, use of strong drugs is unnecessary and often harmful. For the non-disease condition of menopause they are often unnecessary and unwise.

The Value of Using Whole Plants

The modern pharmaceutical industry grew out of the use of herbs for treating specific complaints. The natural chemicals that plants produce to protect themselves from toxins can also be used by humans. In Maharishi Vedic Medicine, a wide variety of plants and mineral substances are used to rebalance the doshas and thereby the whole physiology. In the Ayurvedic pharmacology—called *dravyaguna*—plants, or plant parts are used as they occur in nature, with all their ingredients. Unfortunately, Western pharmacology isolates active ingredients from plants and then usually synthesizes them.

In the early 1800s, a German pharmacist isolated morphine, a pure active ingredient, from the opium plant. This revolutionized the Western medical world but it also created some problems—adverse side effects.

Modern medical science made a mistake when they isolated what they termed "active" ingredients. The scientists believed that all of a plant's desirable properties were in a single compound and all the other compounds "inactive." Using a purified compound instead of the whole plant was thought of as "better."

"The active ingredient approach compromises whatever synergies exist among organic components, which can be significant. The erroneous idea that plants and isolated active principles are equivalent has become fixed dogma in pharmacology and medicine. In general, isolated and refined drugs are much more toxic than their botanical sources, and they lack the natural safeguards present in the whole plant."[2]

Many apparently inactive ingredients have turned out to play significant health-giving roles. Bioflavonoids, a class of molecules found in plants, were once dismissed by researchers. Later researchers found them to have many benefits and to act as antioxidants, anti-inflammatory agents, anti-tumor and anti-allergic agents, to name a few.

Using only the active ingredient and not the whole plant also creates those unwanted side effects that are named in long, hard-to-read lists on every pharmaceutical product. Active ingredients act indiscriminately, not only at the site intended but also at other sites and organs. This is why toxicity arises. "With whole herbs, inactive ingredients are thought to help control the effect at non-target sites."[3]

Vitamins

Both standard Western medicine and practitioners of alternative medicine regard taking vitamins as a means to maintaining good health. Physicians and health professionals prescribe vitamins routinely to their patients with vitamins A, C, and D seeming to be the most popular. However, if the individual constitution is not considered, large doses or unnecessary doses of vitamins may create imbalances in the doshas. Many people who regularly take vitamins and minerals continue to have the same deficiencies for which they are taking supplements because they are unable to properly digest, assimilate and absorb natural or synthetic vitamins. If the physiology is clogged with toxic build-up or the agni (digestive fire) is not adequate, then the vitamins virtually have nowhere to go.

Herbs That Heal

While rebalancing Becky's physiology with practice of the TM technique, rasayanas, proper diet, and lifestyle changes, she remarked how very well she felt. "I hardly have any headaches anymore," she said. "I feel more relaxed while driving. I have more energy and I am, therefore, not consuming as much caffeine. All my problems have improved. I only hope these herbs aren't addictive."

I assured her that Maharishi Ayur-Veda herbal compounds are not addictive, that they are balancing and rejuvenating and that the side benefits are improved health. I explained that because of the holistic way in which they are prepared, they work on the mind and body to improve the whole physiology simultaneously. Ayurveda has long asserted that rasayanas have no side effects because they use the whole plant which within itself produces balance.

Maharishi Vedic Medicine uses rasayanas to stimulate overall health. The term means, "that which supports *rasa*." Rasa is the first of the seven dhatus. It relates to blood plasma and nourishes all the other bodily tissues. Rasayanas also stimulate the production of ojas, the substance that sustains all the dhatus. The herbs in rasayanas are combined in precise proportions and prepared in the traditional Ayurvedic way. This improves the bioavailability of vital nutrients. It also creates synergy—the collective benefit is much greater than that of isolated active ingredients. Or, to put it another way, the effect of the whole is more powerful than the sum of the parts.

At menopause specific rasayanas are used to help balance, strengthen and nourish the hormones, emotions, muscles and bones. They also help with the assimilation and formation of the blood. For example, *Lodhra Bark* and *Sensitive Plant* help nourish the uterus and help balance Apana Vata (responsible for the downward flow of energy), Ranjaka Pitta (responsible for healthy blood and liver function) and Bhrajaka Pitta (responsible for the skin). Other herbs that help nourish the uterus are *Tropical Ficus, Myrrh* and *Silk Cotton Resins.* Combined in the traditional way with other herbs that aid bioavailability, these herbs collectively benefit a woman at menopause.

The ancient texts say that rasayanas promote health by increasing resistance to disease, activating tissue repair mechanisms, and stopping or reversing the deterioration associated with aging. In the *Charaka* texts, it says that rasayanas promote "longevity, memory, intelligence, freedom from disorders, youthfulness, excellence of luster, complexion and voice, optimum strength of physique and sense organs. . . ."

Several months after starting her holistic program that included specific rasayanas for menopause, Becky looked more relaxed and happy. Her comment was, "I am thinking more clearly now. My sleep and concentration, in fact, *everything* is pretty good. I've always been a person who was easily overwhelmed. This has been the anniversary of the death of two family members, which has overwhelmed me in the past. Now I am able to handle it. I do not feel any fear while driving now. That is a remarkable achievement for me."

Free Radicals and Rasayanas as Antioxidants

Research on rasayanas is ongoing. The National Institutes of Health has given grants to study these ancient herbal formulas as antioxidants. To understand the value of studying the effects of antioxidant herbal preparations it is necessary to understand what oxidation does in the body.

Oxygen, which is necessary for life, can also be destructive to the body, causing decay just as it rusts metal. Living in the earth's atmosphere, we continue to survive only because inert nitrogen dilutes oxygen down to 20% of the air we breathe—and the body has developed mechanisms to counter oxygen's destructive effects at levels this low. Oxygen powers the chemical reactions that provide energy for motion, sensation, and thought—for everything that makes possible animal and human life on this planet.

But the oxygen that saturates our cells is also a constant threat to our survival. It mounts a relentless attack that eventually wears down our defenses and destroys our biological machinery. The body gets old because, in large part, oxygen wastes it away. The body suffers from a heart attack, or a stroke, or an outbreak of cancer because oxygen has done its damage. When oxygen combines with hydrogen it produces small molecules called free radicals. These dangerous free radical molecules are also known as oxy radicals. Other atomic and molecular varieties of oxygen are known as reactive oxygen species (ROS). These two terrorists, oxy radicals and ROS, attack DNA, enzymes and proteins, and disrupt normal cell activities.

Diseases Linked to Oxy Radicals and Reactive Oxygen Species

- Cancer
- Heart disease
- Stroke
- Diabetes mellitus
- Arteriosclerosis, atherosclerosis
- Cerebrovascular disease
- Emphysema
- Rheumatoid arthritis

- Osteoporosis
- Sunburn
- Crohn's disease
- Senility
- Ulcers
- Cataracts
- Raynaud's disease
- Aging

Free radicals are not all bad. The immune system cells create oxy radicals and ROS deliberately as weapons to fight bacteria and viruses. Unfortunately, stress, pollution, overexposure to the sun, a diet high in processed foods, and lack of exercise can all cause an overabundance of harmful free radicals.

The body, however, has an anti-free-radical defense system known as antioxidant systems whose job it is to keep oxy radicals and ROS in line. These systems include enzymes, vitamins and other nutrients, including vitamin C and E, beta-carotene, bioflavonoids, and many others. Organic fruits and vegetables are also a good source of antioxidants.

Many free radical researchers feel that to fight free radicals effectively the general levels of all these free radical-fighting nutrients need to be much higher than nutritional experts previously thought. In order to stay healthy the body needs only to strike a proper balance between the number of free radicals generated and the defense and repair mechanisms available.[4]

The most powerful antioxidants in nature are in herbs. When there is the proper mixture of herbs, they can control a large amount of free radicals. So, if on one side, we indulge in activities that create more free radicals, and on the other side, we have enzymes and antioxidants, then there's a balance. But if there is yet more production of free radicals, you have to balance it further; otherwise there will be increased damage.

Here is where rasayanas come in. They are powerful free radical scavengers that help to balance the body. The recipes for these herbal formulations were first discovered thousands of years ago, but over time became lost to the general public or hidden from

India's foreign invaders. However, the formulas were handed down through generations of Ayurvedic physicians called *vaidyas.*

The ancient herbal formulas are completely different from modern drugs.

They are combinations of intact plants or parts of plants, which work as a whole to enrich the human physiology in its entirety. There is no isolation of active ingredients involved as with modern drugs. These rich foods are used as additions to the everyday diet to help promote health and well-being. Rasayanas can easily be eaten and digested.

The History of Rasayanas

With the introduction of Maharishi Vedic Medicine into the world came the rediscovery of the ancient knowledge of rasayanas. At a conference of vaidyas, invited together by Maharishi Mahesh Yogi to discuss what additional knowledge could be made to the modern world, the ancient herbal formula of *amrit kalash* was revealed.

Among the great vaidyas at the conference were Dr. B. D. Triguna, then President of the All-India Ayurvedic Congress, and Director of the National Academy for Ayurveda, Government of India; Dr. Balraj Maharshi, an adviser on Ayurveda to the government of Andhra Pradesh, and a leading expert on *dravyaguna,* the identification and utilization of medicinal plants. Also at the conference was Dr. V. M. Dwivedi, Professor Emeritus, Gujarat Ayurvedic University, and former Vice-Chairman of the Indian Government's Ayurveda Pharmacopoeia Committee. Dr. Dwivedi was one of the few remaining vaidyas in India who was a master of the procedures for creating rasayanas. Among the three of these great and well-respected vaidyas was an immense knowledge of rasayanas.[5]

Balraj Maharshi revealed that he had the formula for amrit kalash, which is an herbal formula that strengthens every cell for optimum health and vitality. He had been told by the wise vaidya who had passed on the formula to him to not reveal it until the time was right to be widely used. Dr. Balraj Maharshi decided that now was the time and that the formula could be scientifically accepted.

The three great vaidyas then worked together, and along with other vaidyas, prepared the mixture in accordance with the ancient standards recorded in the classical Ayurvedic texts. Dr. Triguna also provided another ancient herbal formula that could be used to strengthen the body's immune system. Thus, two separate formulations were provided for amrit kalash. They were named collectively Maharishi Amrit Kalash and are meant to be taken together for maximum effectiveness.

Dr. Triguna's formulation is a nectar herbal fruit concentrate while Dr. Balraj Maharshi's formulation is an herbal tablet. Taken together they create a "super food" that contains 44 herbs and fruits. This combination is a powerful antioxidant—1,000 times more potent than vitamin C or E. It helps the body to defend itself from too many free radicals, which are related to premature aging and disease.

How the rasayanas are prepared is of the utmost importance—a concept not yet grasped by the West. The optimum time to gather an herb—called plant chronobiology—differs at different times of the year since the presence and levels of phytochemicals differ at different times of the year. Therefore, the whole plants are harvested at their peak.

Then the herbs are prepared through a long and careful process of grinding to release their most refined substances and to maximize their ease of digestibility. There is no attempt to isolate individual molecules. Amrit kalash is prepared according to the age-old formula related in the Ayurvedic texts. Twenty-two pounds of raw ingredients, such as whole herbs and fruits, go into the process of making the herbal fruit concentrate alone.

The vaidyas say that the effectiveness of rasayanas comes from the deliberate attempt to maximize synergism. The components help each other move through the digestive system, arrive at the correct cells, penetrate the cell membranes, and keep the cells healthy.

Modern Research on These Ancient Formulas

Much research is performed by or funded by drug companies looking for ways to sell more drugs. If a drug company can synthesize an ingredient, then they can patent it and thus make money from its production.

Nevertheless, there are scientists working at universities worldwide who look at other, natural ways to keep us healthy. Some of the funding for these studies is given by the National Institutes of Health or health organizations in those countries that have no ties to the drug industry. Studies on Maharishi Amrit Kalash, not performed by drug companies, look at its effect on various health issues.

Research is ongoing on rasayanas. Scientists are looking at the effects of rasayanas on numerous problems, including hypertension, types of cancers, depression, pain and aging. To date there are more than 50 modern research studies on amrit kalash.[6] Of course, there have been thousands of years of clinical observations by Ayurvedic practitioners as to the effectiveness of these formulations. Modern studies have found that amrit kalash nourishes the body, mind and spirit by reducing free-radical damage. In four research studies, it significantly boosted the immune response, improved its efficiency, and aided the body's defense system. It also strengthened macrophage cells that kill bacteria.[7]

The Effects of Maharishi Amrit Kalash on Emotions, Depression, Breast Cancer and Aging

The worries that women bring to me at menopause can be greatly reduced or eliminated by incorporating the holistic approaches of Maharishi Vedic Medicine, including the use of rasayanas. Because our modern diet and lifestyles encourage too many harmful free radicals in our bodies, taking the effective free-radical scavenger

MAHARISHI AMRIT KALASH

The Most Effective Antioxidant

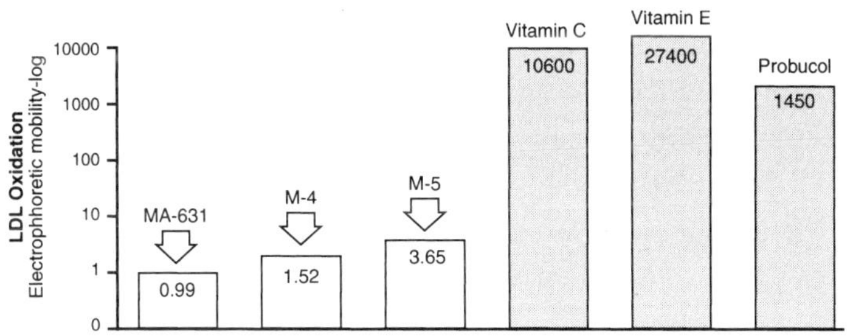

Comparison of Different Anti-Oxidants

MA-631, M-4, M-5 vs. vitamins C, E, and probucol, $p < .0001$

Research shows that Maharishi Amrit Kalash is 1000 times more effective than Vitamin C in scavenging free radicals.

Reference: H.M. Sharma et al., "Inhibition of Human Low-Density Lipoprotein Oxidation in Vitro by Maharishi Amrit Kalash and Maharishi Coffee Substitute" *Pharmacology, Biochemistry and Behavior*, vol. 43 (1992), pp. 1175–1182.

Increased Resistence to Disease

Research shows that Maharishi Amrit Kalash:

- increases immunity
- prevents atherosclerosis by reducing human platelet aggregation
- reduces LDL (bad) cholesterol
- reduces chemical toxicity

References: 1. "Enhanced Lymphoproliferative Response, Macrophage-Mediated Tumor Cell Killing and Nitric Oxide Production after Ingestion of an Ayurvedic Drug (Maharishi Amrit Kalash)," *Biochemical Archives*, vol. 9 (1993), pp. 365–374.
2. H.M. Sharma et al., "Maharishi Amrit Kalash Prevents Human Platelet Aggregation," *Clinica and Terapia Cardiovascolare*, vol. 8, no. 3 (1989), pp. 227–230.
3. A.N. Hanna et al., "Effect of Herbal Mixtures MAK-4 and MAK-5 on Susceptibility of Human LDL to Oxidation, *Complementary Medicine International*, vol. 3, no. 3 (May/June 1996), pp. 28-36.
4. S.C. Bondy, et al., "Antioxidant Preperties of Two Ayurvedic Herbal Preparations (MAK-4 and MAK-5)," *Biochemical Archives*, vol. 10 (1994), pp. 25-31.

Maharishi Amrit Kalash as a means to optimize health, especially at this time in a woman's life, only makes sense.

Here are some of the reported benefits of Maharishi Amrit

Kalash herbal preparations:

- Slows premature aging
- Sharpens mental focus
- Combats stress
- Enhances natural beauty
- Increases alertness
- Reduces fatigue
- Elevates energy levels
- Improves creativity
- Restores inner calm
- Creates mental and physical balance
- Provides a sense of well-being

Maharishi Amrit Kalash and the Emotions

As you already know, the emotions have a powerful effect on the body.

The Vedic texts say that rasayanas enhance psychological well-being. Studies on the effects of Maharishi Amrit Kalash on both psychological mood and biochemical operations in the brain showed that the people using the rasayana had improvements in psychological mood—greater happiness, tranquility, mental clarity, and emotional balance.[8]

Maharishi Amrit Kalash and Depression

A study showed that Maharishi Amrit Kalash interacted with the same receptor on blood platelets as imipramine. Imipramine is a prescription drug given for depression. It binds with a receptor in the brain cells that increases the output of serotonin. Studies have shown that low levels of serotonin relate to such mental health problems as aggression and hostility. High levels of serotonin relate to a stable or exhilarated emotional state. Imipramine, the serotonin trigger, binds not only to brain cells but also to blood platelets, providing another tie between mind and body. This suggests that Maharishi Amrit Kalash might bind to the same receptor in brain cells, since it too interacted with the same receptor on blood platelets as imipramine. This means that taking Maharishi Amrit Kalash would increase serotonin levels and thus psychological mood.[9]

Maharishi Amrit Kalash and Breast Cancer

Studies indicate that cancer may be tied to free radical damage. The effectiveness of taking amrit kalash was studied at The Ohio State University College of Medicine and South Dakota State University in relation to the prevention and regression of breast carcinoma.

The cancer is thought to be a two-step process:

1. an apparently irreversible initiation stage, when alterations occur in the DNA of one or more cells; and
2. a promotion stage, in which the population of initiated cells expands.

Free radicals are active in both of these phases.[10]

In the initiation stage, white blood cells are constantly releasing showers of free radicals that eventually damage the cells' DNA. In the promotion stage, cancer cells generate free radicals and ROS which spread from one area to many areas. There is also evidence that cancerous cells still living in the body produce free radicals and ROS. And aggressive tumor cell populations show increased production of antioxidants, indicating a need to protect themselves against self-generated free radicals.[11]

Both the initiation phase and the promotion phase of breast cancer were studied on laboratory animals given the herbal fruit concentrate formula of Maharishi Amrit Kalash. After 18 weeks, only 25 percent of the animals receiving the formula during the promotion phase showed tumors as compared to 67 percent of the animals in the control group. However, there did not appear to be comparable protection during the initiation phase.[12]

Another experiment was designed using the herbal tablet of Maharishi Amrit Kalash. These results showed 60 percent fewer tumors in the initiation stage and 88 percent fewer tumors in the promotion stage as compared to controls. In addition, in both studies, control animals who had already developed fully formed tumors were given the Maharishi Amrit Kalash diet. In 60 percent of these animals in both studies, the tumors shrank significantly. In roughly half of those that experienced this tumor regression, the tumor disappeared completely.[13]

Chemotherapy

Chemotherapy often destroys cancer cells by producing free radicals. However, free radicals sometime cause new cancers. Maharishi Amrit Kalash has been shown to be effective in reducing the toxic side effects associated with chemotherapy such as vomiting and diarrhea. It also improved sleep, weight and the overall feeling of well-being.[14]

Maharishi Amrit Kalash and Aging

Scientists are always looking for ways to slow down the aging process and extend life. In one study Maharishi Amrit Kalash was fed to 18-month-old mice, which is approximately 50 to 60 years of age in human terms. Even starting at this age, 80 percent of the Maharishi Amrit Kalash group survived to 23 months of age, compared to only 48 percent survival for the control group.[15]

To study the effect of the rasayana on life span, fruit flies, which have a short life-span, were fed the formula. The flies with the Maharishi Amrit Kalash diet lived 70 percent longer than controls.[16] Another study, this time on humans, demonstrated that Maharishi Amrit Kalash's free-radical scavenging ability may rejuvenate cell function, thus improving a complex physical/mental process that seems to deteriorate when we age.

The Use of Herbs and Spices in Maharishi Vedic Medicine

Rasayanas are not the only use of herbs found in the ancient Ayurvedic texts. In general, Maharishi Ayur-Veda uses combinations of herbs which act synergistically to aid the body in healing. But individual herbs are also used, which have specific medical effects. Combinations of herbs and spices are often used to help balance the doshas in different ways. Just as spices have different effects on the physiology, herbs too can be either heating or cooling. Ayurveda also looks at the quality of the herb.

A vaidya can determine what kind of "tastes" the herb or spice has, (bitter, sweet, etc.); its potency (hot or cold); and its aftertaste (bitter, sweet, etc.). The herbs and spices are known for their different qualities and can be used to balance the doshas. For example, fresh ginger root has a pungent taste, a sweet aftertaste and it's hot. It is used to aid digestion and to help balance Vata and Kapha. It has many other uses, including warding off colds and stimulating the appetite. It is useful in its dried form for constipation. It also aids in bioavailability when combined with other herbs.

The effects of herbs are widely studied and have been known for centuries. In spite of this, there has been relatively little research and marketing of natural herbs in the West. Synthesizing herbs and vitamins, however, is being quickly accomplished by pharmaceutical companies. You may have heard advertisements recommending specific brands of natural herbs or natural vitamins because they are "patented," implying that they are better than "unpatented" herbs or vitamins. What it really means is that they have been synthesized in the laboratory. Just because a product says "natural" on the label does not mean that it comes directly from nature.

In the understanding of Maharishi Vedic Medicine, each molecule in an herb is actually an impulse of intelligence, a particular vibration in the underlying field of consciousness.[17] When carefully chosen by experts with the knowledge of the herb's effects, these impulses of intelligence match the impulses of intelligence in different parts of the human body. When the mind and body become out of balance, there are disruptions in the natural sequence that leads from pure intelligence to the complete physiology. Where a sequence is disrupted, disease can occur. The herbal preparations of Maharishi Vedic Medicine provide the correct impulse to reset a particular sequence and the doshas are rebalanced.

Since the body is a self-repairing mechanism, if given the chance and the proper life-supporting ingredients—herbs, herbal combinations and, in fact, all of the approaches of Maharishi Vedic Medicine—the body can stay tuned up and functioning properly for a very long time.

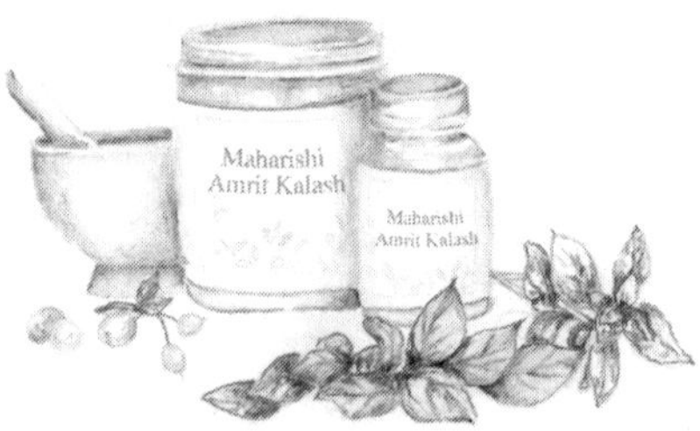

Maharishi Vedic Medicine utilizes a variety of herbal food supplements to enhance the body's resistence to infection and disease.

References

1. Leape, L.L. Error in medicine, *Journal of the American Medical Association.* 272(23), 1851–1857.
2. Guiness, A.E. 1993. *Family Guide to Natural Medicine.* Pleasantville, NY: Reader's Digest Association, Inc., p. 295.
3. Sharma, H. & Clark, C. 1998. *Contemporary Ayurveda.* Philadelphia, PA: Churchill Livingston, p. 76.
4. *Contemporary Ayurveda,* p. 79.
5. *Contemporary Ayurveda,* p. 80.
6. Sharma, H. 1993. *Freedom From Disease.* Toronto, Veda Publishing.

pp. 282–284.

7. *Contemporary Ayurveda*, p. 84.
8. *Freedom From Disease*, p. 166.
9. Hauser, T., Walton, K.G, Glaser, J., Wallace, R.K. 1988 (Nov. 14). *Naturally occurring ligand inhibits binding of [3H] imipramine to high affinity receptors.* Paper presented at the 18th Annual Meeting of the Society for Neuroscience, p. 244 (abstract).
10. Fischer, S.M., Floyd, R.A. & Copeland, E.S. 1988. Oxy radicals in carcinogenesis. Workshop report from the Division of Research Grants, NIH. *Cancer Research,* 48, 3662–3887.
11. Borunov, E.V., Smirnova, L.P., Shchepetkin, I.A., Lankin, V.Z. & Vasiliev, N.V. 1989. High antioxidative enzyme activity in tumors is a factor making the immune system "out of control." *Bulletin of Exp. Bio and Med,* 107(4), 530–532.
12. Sharma, H.M., Dwivedi, C., Satter, B.C. & Abou-Issa, H. 1991. Antineoplastic properties of Maharishi Amrit Kalash, an Ayurvedic food supplement, against 7, 12-dimethylbenz(a)anthracene-induced mammary tumors in rats. *Journal of Research and Education in Indian Medicine,* 10(3), 1–8.
13. Sharma H.M et al., 1991.
14. Misra, N.C., Sharma, H.M., Chaturvedi, A. et al. 1994. Antioxidant adjuvant therapy using a natural herbal mixture (MAK) during intensive chemotherapy; reduction in toxicity: A prospective study of 62 patients. Proceedings of the XVI International Cancer Congress. Monduzzi, Bologna, pp. 3099–3102.
15. Fields, J.Z., Eftekhari, E., Hagen, J.F., Wichlinski, L.J. & Schneider, R.H. 1991. Anti-aging and oxygen free radical (ORF) scavenging effects of an anti-carinogenic natural product, Maharishi Amrit Kalash. *Journal of the Federation of AM Societies for Experimental Biology,* 5(6), A1735 (abstract).
16. Fields, J.Z. et al. 1991.
17. Sharma, H. & Clark, C. *Contemporary Ayurveda*, p. 93.

Chapter Fourteen

Maharishi Vedic Medicine—A Closer Look

As you have seen, there are many ways to create balance in the physiology. These approaches to health are collectively known as Maharishi Vedic Medicine. Maharishi Vedic Medicine, based on total knowledge of Natural Law (Veda), has as its fundamental principle that in order to prevent sickness and disease, the inner intelligence of every aspect of the physiology must be maintained in its full alertness, its full vitality.

This inner intelligence consists of the fundamental structures of Natural Law—the 40 aspects of Veda and the Vedic Literature—which govern human physiology and the whole universe. The profound and practical application of this knowledge to health helps to bring all aspects of individual life into harmony with Natural Law—the basis for maintaining health and creating a disease-free society.

Remember, the body is a self-repairing system. When an influence is introduced that resonates with the body's underlying intelligence, the body automatically responds and adapts or corrects itself to restore inner harmony. The more you incorporate these fundamental approaches into your surroundings, the more balanced your life will be.

It isn't that stresses and strains will suddenly disappear; but by using these techniques you will be able to handle life's problems more easily without being caught up in them. Not only does this relate to the hormonal fluctuations you may experience at menopause but it relates to the normal fluctuations of life.

Fortunately, you may already be using many of these approaches to health. This, then, can be a common-sense reminder to use the tools you already have, or it can give you more of an understanding of how these techniques work.

The first tool is the Transcendental Meditation technique which has been briefly discussed. There is an inseparable connection between the unmanifest field of consciousness and all the manifest levels of the physiology. That is why Maharishi Vedic Medicine uses the natural approach of consciousness, the Transcendental Meditation program, as its primary tool. It also handles health from the more expressed levels of health—physiology, behavior, and environment—through natural daily and seasonal routines; healthy, balanced diet; proper exercise; and herbal preparations. It also handles health from the field of knowledge—from the knowledge of balance—and the knowledge of the inseparable connection between consciousness and its expression, the physiology.

Your Environment

A person's surroundings reflect on the inner well-being of the person who created it. A healthy, well-centered woman will have a healthy, well-centered environment. That environment will, in turn, help her to be healthy and well-centered.

Accordingly, where you live and how you live has an effect on your health. The term "sick building syndrome" is a very real phenomenon. By using unhealthy types of insulation, poor ventilation, restricted access to natural light, synthetic furniture and improper orientation of the building, health and happiness can be affected.

The ancient architectural discipline of *Sthapatya Veda* uses building techniques that maximize health and put you in harmony with the processes of nature. It considers orientation, light, ventilation, natural building materials and design techniques that have a beneficial effect on the dwellers.

Maharishi Sthapatya Veda design comprises a series of timeless principles that describe the fine mechanisms whereby nature creates proportion and shapes objects, such as planets, stars, trees and human bodies. These principles can be used by architects in creating homes and offices. These principles are like the DNA of architecture.

Landscaping or natural settings are also in the realm of Maharishi Sthapatya Veda design. Modern research on the effects of your surroundings in relation to landscaping has compared patients whose hospital room windows looked out on a grove of deciduous trees versus those patients whose windows looked out upon a building. The patients with the natural view had a shorter hospital stay and a more positive post-surgical recovery.[1]

The desire to have a safe and healthy home is one of the most fundamental of human desires. Maharishi Sthapatya Veda design fills that desire. (See the Index for more information.)

The Senses

A pleasing environment can appeal to the senses which, in turn, creates an impact on your physiology. The senses bring in information from the outside that can affect the balance of the doshas and dhatus, and thus affect your health. According to Vedic thought, the ego, intellect, mind, and the senses are sequential manifestations of consciousness. Every sense has a direct channel to the brain and, through the limbic system and other channels, affects the whole physiology. Because of this, Maharishi Vedic Medicine has methods that appeal to the senses, thus balancing them and through them, balancing your whole mind-body system.

Of the five senses: hearing (ears), feeling (skin), seeing (eyes), tasting (tongue) and smelling (nose), two have been discussed—feeling and tasting. The sense of touch or feeling can be satisfied through self-massage and rejuvenation massage at Maharishi Ayur-Veda Health Centers. Satisfying the sense of taste has been discussed through the use of the six tastes in your diet. Satisfying the other senses is easy to incorporate into your life through sound therapy, aroma therapy and color therapy.

Healing through Hearing or Sound Therapy

Sounds plays a central role in Maharishi Vedic Medicine. It is well known around the world that sounds and music can affect the physiology. Modern physics states that the infinite number of elements in the universe, at their fundamental basis, are simply frequency or sounds. Every type of matter has a characteristic frequency at which it normally vibrates. This is true as well for cells, tissues, organs and the entire physiology. As human beings we are all made up of the sounds of nature and vibrate within ourselves and within our environment. Sometimes we get out of tune. Maharishi Vedic Medicine incorporates the use of sounds on many different levels to help restore health and balance to the physiology.

Many studies have shown how music affects the body. The external vibrations produced by music in the environment have been shown to alter inner vibrations at the molecular and pre-molecular level. Music can change pulse rate, circulation, and blood pressure. There can be an increase or decrease in metabolism, muscular energy and respiration rate.[2] Music can help alleviate acute pain and decrease the use of pain medication.[3] It is almost certain that the external vibrations produced by music in the environment alter inner vibrations at the molecular level. The melody and rhythmic structure of music is metabolized through the limbic system, which helps regenerate (or agitate) the body.

Sound therapy can be understood in terms of the primordial sounds of creation resetting the spontaneous sequential order which lies at the basis of the physiology. By utilizing these primordial sounds of nature as part of therapy, this sequential order of creation can be reset to its proper value, reestablishing orderliness of the entire physiology.

Another way of thinking about it is to think of using sound

therapy as a way of tuning yourself up, just as one tunes a guitar. The guitar player hits a tuning fork, sets the base of the tuning fork on the body of the guitar, and the guitar begins to resonate in that tone. The guitar player then adjusts the string to match the pitch of the tuning fork. The main difference here is that whereas the guitar player has to do something to tune the string, the physiology automatically responds to the Vedic sounds to reset its functioning to a state of better health.

By listening to the sounds of the Veda, one enlivens basic frequencies within consciousness. Individual awareness is brought in tune with those fundamental fluctuations of the laws of nature. This experience brings increased balance to the psychophysiology, the mind-body metabolizes the most basic laws of nature and "retunes" itself back to health.[4]

Maharishi Gandharva Veda℠ Music

Gandharva Veda's theme is "life is music" and it is the name for the traditional classical music of India. Maharishi Gandharva Veda is a sophisticated and precise science of Vedic melodies that have a positive effect on the balance of the doshas.

In Maharishi Vedic Medicine it is understood that the doshas can be aggravated or balanced by rhythms and melodies. The Ayurvedic texts list specific times of the day for playing of different melodies, or *ragas*, of Gandharva Veda. One type of raga can help create energy and dynamism for activity during the day, while another creates relaxation in the evening.

Listening to the proper raga at the proper time of day helps smooth the natural transitions from one cycle of day to another. They attune the body and mind to the proper biological rhythms. Also, specific ragas can be prescribed by physicians trained in Maharishi Ayur-Veda to help balance specific doshas and subdoshas.

Maharishi Gandharva Veda music tapes or CDs can be played in your home to create a soothing atmosphere. You can play the music even when you are not home, because the music will have a balancing influence within the home. When you return home you will return to this wonderful atmosphere of harmony. (For more information see the Index.)

Maharishi Vedic SoundsSM

Particular sounds, known as Maharishi Vedic Sounds, have a positive effect on mind and body. The pronunciation, melody and rhythmic pattern of these sounds have been preserved as the basic source material of the Vedic tradition in the *Ṛk Veda* and three companion sources, *Sama Veda, Yajur Veda,* and *Atharva Veda.* According to the ancient texts, the sound patterns preserved in these collections reflect the primordial vibrations at the basis of nature.

According to neurophysiologist Tony Nader, M.D., Ph.D., in his book *Human Physiology; Expression of Veda and Vedic Literature,* "Our physiology is continuously performing millions of tasks to maintain order and balance in its functioning, to allow growth and evolution to occur, and to bring about increasing achievement and fulfillment.

"The perfect order displayed in the human physiology and throughout the universe is based on Laws of Nature that have been studied by modern science for more than 150 years. Profound insights into the ancient Vedic Literature of India brought to light by His Holiness Maharishi Mahesh Yogi have guided the recent discovery that the laws that construct the human mind and body are the same as those that give structure to the syllables, verses, chapters and books of the Vedic Literature. Moreover, the sounds of the syllables, verses and hymns of the Vedic Literature are the frequencies whose vibrations enliven specific aspects of the physiology.

"Just as the structure of the various branches of Vedic Literature correspond to specific structures in the physiology, the sounds of those verses also contain the same corresponding intelligence. Thus recitations of the sounds of the Vedic Literature in their proper sequence will resonate with the same anatomic structures to which they correspond. Their specific sequence will also enliven a specific sequence of neuronal physiological activity. This will induce the physiology to function according to its original and perfect design. Any imperfections in the form of blocks, stress, lack or excess of activity, or abnormal connections between the various components of the physiology, will be disfavored by reading or listening to the specific aspect of Veda and the Vedic Literature that corresponds to that area of the physiology which is dysfunctional."[5]

One particular branch of Vedic Literature, Sama Veda, is recommended "without prescription" as sounds that everyone can listen to in order to restore balanced functioning of the sensory systems and perception apparatus.

Studies at The Ohio State University by Dr. Hari Sharma and colleagues found that Sama Veda decreased human cancer cell growth in laboratory experiments. The study stated, "The process of carcinogenesis has been shown to change cellular vibrations, and it is known that normal DNA has low-frequency vibrations, so perhaps the low-frequency vibrations of Sama Veda inhibited growth of the cancer cells."[6]

Traditionally, Sama Veda is played for a few minutes before going to bed.

Aroma Therapy

As we breathe, odor-bearing molecules activate receptors in the nose. These translate into nerve impulses, which reach the olfactory bulbs in the brain. These bulbs are directly connected to the limbic area of the brain surrounding the hypothalamus, which processes emotions, and to the hippocampus, an area of the brain responsible for memory. Certain aromas will trigger certain memories, such as when the smell of baking bread instantly takes you to your mother's kitchen.

Aroma therapy has suddenly been "rediscovered" in the United

States. But sometimes the knowledge of how aromas can heal is not put into effect. Going to the store and buying a "watermelon-scented" aroma or a "rum-flavored" aroma is not going to help balance your doshas.

Maharishi Vedic Medicine uses a wide range of aromas, usually floral or herbal essences, precisely calibrated to pacify specific doshas or subdoshas. They are used in treatments at Maharishi Ayur-Veda Health Centers or can be used at home. These Therapeutic Aroma™ scents can do wonders for your mind and physiology as well as create a welcoming and soothing atmosphere in your home. Therapeutic Aroma scents use the finest and freshest ingredients.

Most often the aroma oils are diffused through the air by putting drops of oil in aroma pots or aroma diffusers. If you need to balance your physiology for weight loss, then an aroma oil with invigorating scents such as ginger, orange, lemon, fennel or grapefruit will stimulate your metabolism. Aroma oils are used for everything from enlivening to calming the environment.

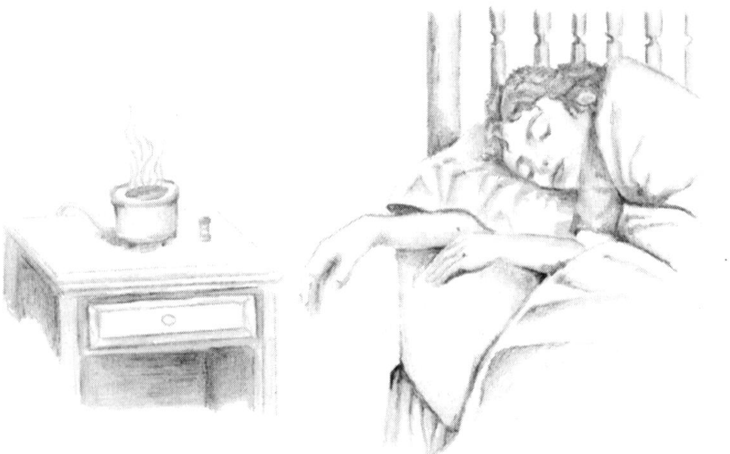

A soothing therapeutic aroma oil blend will help you sleep and restore balance all night long.

Color Therapy

Just as sound has an effect on the physiology, so do different frequencies of light. When white light splits into different frequencies, it produces separate bands of color: red, orange, yellow, green, blue, and purple—the colors of the rainbow. Because the basic colors of the rainbow are correlated with the dhatus and the doshas, their vibratory energy may be used to help establish balance in your home. For example, Maharishi Ayur-Veda Health Centers use soft soothing pastels as part of their decor.

Maharishi Jyotish Program

Jyotish is a science of understanding and predicting future trends in an individual's (or a company's, or a country's) life. With reference to health concerns, it is the mathematical approach to diagnosis, identification of future problems or illness, along with prescriptions and programs for prevention and cure. Sometimes known as Maharishi Vedic Astrology℠, the Maharishi Jyotish program is a tool for the evaluation of the environmental influences that may affect your health. The basis of understanding the Maharishi Jyotish program is understanding the spontaneous sequential order inherent in creation. By knowing any one point in this order, one can automatically know all events that have come before and what will follow.

Trained experts in the Maharishi Jyotish program (*jyotishis*) use precise mathematical calculations to take into account important aspects of the environment, including planets and stars. These calculations yield information about the health of an individual. They can also be used to predict future health problems. Maharishi Vedic Medicine uses the Maharishi Jyotish program to foresee health problems so that preventative measures can be used in diverting them.

All impressions and actions from the past as well as their ultimate result are printed in the blueprint of life, the genetic code of DNA. The Maharishi Jyotish program contains the knowledge of what the DNA will produce on which day, thereby giving complete knowledge of the whole physiological reality contained in the genetic code. In this way the Maharishi Jyotish program makes a woman the master of her own destiny.

Maharishi Yagya℠ Program

Modern physicists say that there are mathematically describable laws of nature that structure creation—a "cosmic code" that is like the DNA for the universe. Maharishi explains that the complex sound patterns in the ancient texts Ṛk Veda and other Vedic texts comprise this cosmic code.

The Maharishi Yagya program involves *pandits* who know how to perform various sequences from these Vedic texts. Information is carried by pronunciation, pitch, sequence, and rhythmic pattern. Choice of a particular performance, or *yagya,* to be undertaken is based on the calculations of the Maharishi Jyotish program, so that yagyas can be used to correct imbalances that have not yet manifested.

Here's an example: perhaps in your Maharishi Jyotish reading there is an indication of ill health or some other imbalance that may come up in your life. Having a Maharishi Yagya performance can correct this imbalance so that you never have to experience the ill health or other problem. It's like a rewrite of your life's story before you get to that part of the book.

Maharishi Gemstones and Metals

A Maharishi jyotishi can make recommendations on what type of gems you should wear based on the findings of your Maharishi Jyotish reading. These gems correspond to what planetary influence you wish to strengthen. Since subtle structures of all things, even small gemstones, reflect the same laws of nature, the jyotishi can use specific gemstones to help balance the subtle influences of the sun, moon and planets. To be effective, the gem must be worn directly against the skin, either around the neck or on a specific finger, and must be the specific karat size recommended by the jyotishi.

The metals gold, silver, iron and copper are all known to have specific effects. A gold or silver setting will be recommended by a jyotishi to promote either energy or calmness.

Sometimes a physician trained in Maharishi Ayur-Veda will make a specific recommendation to drink water in the morning that has been standing overnight in a copper drinking glass. Copper helps with excess Kapha and is considered good for the lymphatic system.

Maharishi Vedic Vibration Technology℠

Here is the basic principle of Maharishi Vedic Vibration Technology: if all matter, including the body, is sound waves, then anyone who knows how to use sounds should be able to influence the body. This is exactly what the experts in Maharishi Vedic Vibration Technology do. They use specific sounds to influence specific areas of the body to transform disorder into orderliness, disease into health.

These sounds of Veda are the intelligence that structures the human physiology. The sounds are used in Maharishi Vedic Vibration Technology to enliven the orderly functioning of the physiology, and thereby relieve pain without drugs or surgery or any other invasive therapies. (See the Index for the location of experts in Maharishi Vedic Vibration Technology.)

What to Expect from a Maharishi Ayur-Veda Health Center

A Maharishi Ayur-Veda Health Center can provide you with all of these approaches to health at once. A Maharishi Ayur-Veda Health Center is designed using Maharishi Sthapatya Veda design techniques. All the senses are taken care of through the use of color, music and aromas in the rooms and throughout the building. The treatments use the proper herbs and aromas recommended by the health center's physician who has been trained in Maharishi Ayur-Veda.

The health center's Guest Service staff can help you make a Maharishi Jyotish program appointment, get you in touch with an architect trained in Maharishi Sthapatya Veda design, and give you the latest information on the knowledge of Maharishi Vedic Medicine.

Maharishi Ayur-Veda Health Centers offer comprehensive programs to enliven the body's own inner intelligence to prevent disease and promote good health.

Maharishi Vedic Approach to Health *Consultations*

It is recommended that these consultations be taken initially for the treatment of chronic ailments and imbalances. Once you have gained positive health, they can be taken seasonally or at least twice a year as a preventive measure. During these consultations, the physician will confer with an expert in Maharishi Vedic Medicine. The purpose of this consultation is to allow the physician to determine any imbalances in the system.

The physician then makes recommendations based on the Maharishi Vedic Medicine program to enliven the inner intelligence of the body and help restore balance to the system. Recommendations may be given for diet, daily routine and herbal supplements.

Purification and Rejuvenation Programs

The purification and rejuvenation programs aim at eliminating accumulated impurities in the physiology and restoring balance before any imbalance manifests as disease.

Impurities accumulate in the body from stress and strain, unhealthy diet and behavior, aging, environmental pollution and other factors. These impurities prevent the free flow of intelligence in the physiology, hinder proper digestion, and obstruct the channels of circulation and communication in the body.

The purification and rejuvenation programs available at Maharishi Ayur-Veda Health Centers gently and effectively cleanse the body of accumulated toxins and help restore balance and integrated functioning to the whole physiology, thereby promoting vitality, long life and the prevention of disease.

Initial scientific research on these programs has shown improved cardiovascular functioning, improved appetite and digestion, increased vitality, increased stamina and improved mental clarity.

Program for Individuals with Chronic Disorders

Maharishi Vedic Medicine offers to reestablish balance between the body and its own inner intelligence through Vedic knowledge and its applications. Based on this knowledge, Maharishi Ayur-Veda Health Centers offer comprehensive programs for individuals with chronic disorders.

To participate in the Program for Individuals with Chronic Disorders, applicants complete a specially designed questionnaire related specifically to their health concern. The information on the completed questionnaire is evaluated by a physician who also consults with an additional expert in Maharishi Vedic Medicine. The physician then designs an individually tailored program during a personal consultation with the client. If you suffer from a chronic problem or disorder, contact a Maharishi Ayur-Veda Health Center about this program.

Maharishi RasayanaSM ***Program***

The Maharishi Rasayana program is for prevention, rejuvenation, and holistic well-being of mind and body. It is for healthy people or those who have only minor health problems.

The Maharishi Rasayana program makes use of the different aspects of Maharishi Vedic ScienceSM to allow participants to enliven the Veda (Natural Law) in their own physiology. Maharishi Vedic Medicine recommends a complete rejuvenation program once a year.

The goal of the program is to enable life to progress towards perfect health, without accumulation of the imbalances that express themselves as disease and aging. The Maharishi Rasayana Program is offered in blocks of 40, 30, 20, and 10 days.

This ancient technology is being introduced to the world at this time based on the descriptions of the benefits that appear in the Veda and Vedic Literature.

Some Maharishi Ayur-Veda Health Centers also offer Royal Skin Rejuvenation programs in addition to regular rejuvenation programs.

Maharishi Ayur-Veda Health Centers use the complete knowledge of Natural Law available in the 40 aspects of Veda and the Vedic Literature—the 40 qualities of Natural Law—which have recently been discovered as the basis of the 40 aspects of human physiology.

This discovery by Dr. Nader has been achieved on the basis of more than 30 years of scientific research in physiology and 37 years of discoveries in the field of consciousness by Maharishi Mahesh Yogi. This discovery demonstrates that the total potential of Natural Law is available to everyone as the inner intelligence of his or her own body. These Maharishi Vedic Medicine health programs aim at utilizing this inner intelligence—the intelligence of Natural Law —to enliven the body's own self-repair and balancing mechanisms, and to promote good health.

As a result, thought, behavior, tastes, and tendencies become more integrated and balanced, and spontaneously more in harmony with Natural Law, which is the basis of good health.

I have sent many women to Maharishi Ayur-Veda Health Centers and they report remarkable results in both body and mind. I highly recommend you visit a Maharishi Ayur-Veda Health Center on a regular basis.

References

1. Ulrich, R. 1984. Views through a window may influence recovery from surgery. *Science,* 224, 420–421.
2. McClelland, D.C. 1979. Music in the operating room. *Journal of the Association of Operating Room Nurses,* 29(2), 252–260.
3. Cook, J.D. 1981. The therapeutic use of music: A literature review. *Nursing Forum,* 20(3), 252–266.
4. Oliver, L.H. & Willbanks, S.E. 1999. Sound health. *The Raj Healthy News.*
5. Nader, T. 1995. *Human Physiology: Expression of Veda and the Vedic Literature.* Vlodrop, Holland: Maharishi Vedic University, p. vii, 200–201.
6. Sharma, H.M., Kauffman, E.M. & Stephens, R.E. 1996. Effect of different sounds on growth of human cancer cell lines in vitro. *Alternative Therapies in Clinical Practice,* 3, 25–32.

CHAPTER FIFTEEN

Golden Transition—Feeling Fabulous with Maharishi Vedic Medicine

Menopause marks the beginning of a true woman of wisdom, a transition into a deeper level of spiritual, mental and physical balance. For most women, the symptoms of menopause last for a relatively short time. Eating correctly, exercising, and making other positive lifestyle changes will help you feel great and live a long, healthy life after menopause. It's the decisions you make on a day-to-day basis that determine how healthy you are.

The purpose of writing this book is so you will have a general understanding of Maharishi Vedic Medicine. It is not meant as a self-diagnostic tool as, without specific recommendations from a physician trained in Maharishi Ayur-Veda, you might delay the path of healing. The role of such a physician is to simplify the knowledge and the suggestions made in this book, so that a lot of guess work, trial and error is eliminated on your part and the path is clear and quick for rapid recovery.

The Rest of Your Life

You've learned a lot about the difference between how Western medicine views menopause as a disease and how Maharishi Vedic Medicine views it as a life transition. According to modern science, "health" is a state of "absence of disease." According to the holistic approach of Maharishi Vedic Medicine, health is a state of perfect mental and physical balance, where the full range of consciousness is available and the lifespan is long and healthy.

The Vedic tradition understands that nature is not fundamentally objective. It is not based on material objects. Rather, the most fundamental reality is completely subjective—an unbounded and eternal field of pure, abstract intelligence or consciousness. Consciousness is that which is most intimate to our experience—that which lies beneath thought and feeling. When the mind settles down through the Transcendental Meditation technique, it becomes identified with this pure field of consciousness. This experience is considered by Maharishi Vedic Medicine to be necessary for creating ideal health.

You've also learned that the three doshas, Vata, Pitta, and Kapha, are the fundamental controllers of the physiology. Diet, behavior, perceptions and your surrounding environment all alter the doshic balance and have a significant and specific effect upon your physiology. Imbalances and impurities make you forget your wholeness and an imbalance of the doshas causes discomfort or disease.

When the doshas are in balance, freedom from discomfort and disease is ensured. When the doshas are balanced, health is balanced. The main purpose of Maharishi Vedic Medicine is to keep the doshas, dhatus and malas in balance. Balance is the natural state of life.

For the doshas to be perfectly balanced, consciousness must be fully developed. Transcendental Consciousness is the non-changing, eternal field that forms the basis of perfect health. Maharishi Vedic Medicine brings pure knowledge to the world family, thus reestablishing immortal values of life in every phase of mortal values.

Life is a combination of body, senses, mind and consciousness. Life established in perfect balance means perfect health. Maharishi Vedic Medicine takes the individual as a whole and seeks to reestablish harmony between all the constituents of life. The overall purpose of this system of health care is to develop the highest levels of human functioning in both body and mind.

The definition from the ancient texts of a healthy person is "one whose doshas are in balance, whose appetite is good, whose dhatus are functioning normally, whose malas are in balance, and whose body, mind and senses remain full of bliss."

Proceed One Step at a Time

The knowledge contained in the ancient texts of Ayur-Veda is vast. Where does one begin? Making changes in your daily routine, such as rising early or practicing Maharishi Yoga asanas and the TM technique is a good way to start. Changing your diet and exercise habits will improve your well-being remarkably. You don't have to add everything at once (although if you have a lot of that Pitta drive in your physiology you will think that you *have* to). Small additions will be much better than an all-or-nothing approach.

You are here to enjoy, not to be restricted or uncomfortable. Enjoy life and be happy. Success in anything comes from being happy. Be happy, healthy and let all love flow from your heart.

Remember Who You Really Are and What You Can Really Do

Practice the Transcendental Meditation technique to help you make the right decisions. Your body is a vehicle that takes you toward enlightenment.

Having a good daily routine, which includes the Transcendental Meditation technique, reestablishes your connection to the rhythms of nature that helps you to prevent discomfort or disease in life. Be regular in your new routine.

Abstain from immoderate behavior, even little things like hurrying. Do nothing in excess.

Be self controlled.

Maintain cleanliness of yourself and your environment. This means clear out the ama from your physiology.

Keep the company of the wise. Devote yourself to knowledge and higher states of consciousness.

Develop faith in your life. Your intellect alone can't ensure your progress. Intellect and faith together provide an anchor for greater accomplishment.

Just remember, you choose everything in your life. You always have a choice. Your life unfolds in a sequential pattern. Once you make a choice, you have to deal with the appropriate consequences. You have control over the choice. Choose wisely.

See the wholeness in everything. You are not separate or isolated.

Speak truthfully but sweetly. Abstain from finding fault in yourself or in others. Do not speak ill of others.

Be charitable. Give time and attention to others and to yourself.

This time of personal, positive change can, and should, bring on more change, not only for you, but for your world. So many things in the world need changing and we women at this time of our lives can bring about those changes. World hunger, wars, pollution, homelessness, child abuse, abused women, to name a few, are all issues that we should be able to eliminate in our lifetime.

My recommendation: take care of yourself first, then let's all get together and take care of the world.

APPENDIX

Information Sources on Maharishi Vedic Medicine and Related Programs

HOW TO LOCATE A PHYSICIAN TRAINED IN MAHARISHI VEDIC MEDICINE

Contact your nearest Maharishi Vedic University, College, School, or Center, or one of the Maharishi Ayur-Veda Health Centers (see additional information later in this Appendix).

To contact Kumuda Reddy, M.D.:

11212 Edson Park Place, Rockville, MD 20852
phone: 301-770-0610 or 877-589-0590
Web site: www.allhealthyfamily.com

HOW TO LOCATE A TEACHER OF THE *TRANSCENDENTAL MEDITATION* TECHNIQUE

Call toll-free 888-LEARN-TM (888-532-7686)
or see web site: www.tm.org

WHERE TO ORDER *MAHARISHI AYUR-VEDA* TEAS AND HERBAL FORMULAS

In the United States

Maharishi Ayur-Veda Products International, Inc. — 800-255-8332 or 719-260-5500
P.O. Box 49667
Colorado Springs, CO 80949-9667
Web site: www.mapi.com

In Canada

Maharishi Ayur-Veda Products Canada
Web site: www.all-veda.com

CENTERS OFFERING PROGRAMS IN MAHARISHI VEDIC MEDICINE

In the United States

Maharishi Vedic Vibration Technology — 800-431-9680
Instant Relief℠ program — Fax: 603-588-2115
E-mail: relief@mavf.org
Web site: www.VedicVibration.com

The Raj — 800-248-9050 or 641-472-9580
Fairfield, Iowa
Web site: www.theraj.com

The Heavenly Mountain Clinic — 877-890-8600
Boone, North Carolina

Maharishi Vedic Medical Center — 301-770-5690
Bethesda, Maryland — Fax: 301-770-5694
Web site: www.mvc-bethesda.org

In Canada

Maharishi Ayur-Veda College — 800-575-5472 or 819-837-0772
Waterville, Quebec
E-mail: cvmaha@sympatico.ca

Maharishi Ayur-Veda College — 613-565-2030
Paterson House, Ottawa, Ontario — Fax: 613-565-6546
E-mail: mavcott@istar.ca

More information is available at web sites:
www.Maharishi-medical.com
www.vedic-health.com

THE *MAHARISHI VEDIC ASTROLOGY* AND *MAHARISHI YAGYA* PROGRAMS IN THE UNITED STATES AND CANADA

Maharishi Vedic Astrology program (seminars and consultations)	800-888-5797
Maharishi Vedic Astrology and	800-483-2234
Maharishi Yagya programs	or 603-588-4235
E-mail: usayagya@Maharishi.net	Fax: 603-588-4249
Fairfield, Iowa, office	641-472-5603

More information is available at the web site:
www.Maharishi.org

THE *MAHARISHI STHAPATYA VEDA* PROGRAM

In response to the urgent worldwide need for people to have ideal working and living environments, Maharishi Global Construction, L.L.C. was established to offer consulting services in Maharishi Sthapatya Veda design principles to architects, designers and builders. Maharishi Global Construction is currently building Maharishi Vedic Centers and Maharishi Vedic Medical Centers around the United States.

In the United States:

Maharishi Global Construction, L.L.C.	641-472-9605
500 North Third Street, Suite 110	Fax: 641-472-9083
Fairfield, IA 52556	
E-mail: reception@MGC-Vastu.com	

In Canada:

Maharishi Global Construction	613-565-8525
E-mail: MGC-can@ottawa.com	Fax: 613-565-6546

More information is available at the website:
www.Vedahouse.com

MAHARISHI OPEN UNIVERSITY

This global university delivers the total knowledge of Natural Law via a network of eight satellites to students, working adults, and retired people in every country.

Web site: www.MOU.org

MAHARISHI VEDIC UNIVERSITIES, COLLEGES, SCHOOLS, AND CENTERS

Maharishi Vedic Universities, Colleges, Schools, and Centers are located in most major cities in the United States and in Canada. If you are unable to find a listing from your local telephone directory, or from directory assistance, call toll-free 888-532-7686, or see the following web site: www.Maharishi.org.

HEALTH EDUCATION SHORT COURSES FOR THE WHOLE POPULATION

These 16-hour courses are available at Maharishi Vedic Universities, Colleges and Schools. Full descriptions of these courses can be found at the following web site: www.Maharishi.org.

1. Human Physiology: Expression of Veda and the Vedic Literature
2. Good Health through Prevention
3. The Maharishi Yoga Program
4. Self-Pulse Reading Course for Prevention
5. Diet, Digestion and Nutrition
6. Maharishi Vedic Astrology Overview
7. Maharishi Vedic Architecture

DEGREE PROGRAMS

Bachelor's degree program in Maharishi Vedic Medicine and doctoral degree program in Physiology with specialization in Maharishi Vedic Medicine:

Maharishi University of Management 641-472-4600
College of Maharishi Vedic Medicine
Fairfield, IA 52557
E-mail: admissions@mum.edu
Web site: www.mum.edu/cmvm

Two-year doctor training program; A.A. degree available for beginning students (curriculum authorized by the Commission on Higher Education for the Board of Education for the State of New Mexico):

Maharishi College of Vedic Medicine 505-830-0435
2721 Arizona Street, NE Fax: 505-830-0538
Albuquerque, NM 87110

RECOMMENDED BOOKS

Books by Maharishi Mahesh Yogi

Life Supported by Natural Law. Washington, D.C.: Age of Enlightenment Press, 1986.

Maharishi Forum of Natural Law and National Law for Doctors. India: Age of Enlightenment Publications, 1995.

Maharishi Mahesh Yogi on the Bhagavad-Gita: A New Translation and Commentary, Chapters 1-6. New York: Penguin Books, 1973.

Maharishi Vedic University: Introduction. India: Age of Enlightenment Publications, 1995.

Science of Being and Art of Living. New York: Penguin Books, 1995.

Scientific Research on* Maharishi Ayur-Veda *Health Care

Scientific Research on Maharishi's Transcendental Meditation and TM-Sidhi Program: Collected Papers, Volumes 1–6, available through Maharishi University of Management Press, Press Distribution, DB 1155, Fairfield, Iowa 52557.

Scientific Research on the Maharishi Transcendental Meditation and TM-Sidhi Programs: A Brief Summary of 500 Studies. Fairfield, Iowa: Maharishi University of Management Press, 1996.

Other Books

Nader, Tony, M.D., Ph.D. *Human Physiology: Expression of Veda and the Vedic Literature.* Vlodrop, The Netherlands: Maharishi Vedic University Press, 1994.

Denniston, Denise. *The TM Book: How to Enjoy the Rest of Your Life.* Fairfield, Iowa: Fairfield Press, 1986.

Marcus, Jay. *The Crime Vaccine: How to End the Crime Epidemic.* Baton Rouge, Louisiana: Claitor's Publishing Division, Inc., 1996.

O'Connell, David, and Charles N. Alexander. *Self Recovery: Treating Addictions Using Transcendental Meditation and Maharishi Ayur-Veda.* New York: Haworth Press, 1994.

Roth, Robert. *Maharishi Mahesh Yogi's Transcendental Meditation.* New York: Donald I. Fine, 1994.

Sharma, Hari, M.D. *Freedom from Disease: How to Control Free Radicals, a Major Cause of Aging and Disease.* Toronto: Veda Publishing, 1993.

Wallace, R. Keith. *The Neurophysiology of Enlightenment.* Fairfield, Iowa: Maharishi International University Press, 1986.

Wallace, R. Keith. *The Physiology of Consciousness.* Fairfield, Iowa: Maharishi International University Press, 1993.

These books and others are available from

Maharishi University of Management Press 800-831-6523
Press Distribution DB 1155
Fairfield, Iowa 52557
E-mail: mumpress@mum.edu
Web site: www.mum.edu/press/welcome

A selection of books is also available from Maharishi Ayur-Veda Products (see information above).

GLOSSARY

abhyanga Ayurvedic oil massage

agni digestive fire; also the element of fire generally (see ***mahabhuta***, ***bhutagni***, ***dhatu agni***, and ***jatharagni***)

akasha the element of space (see ***mahabhuta***)

ama the sticky, bad-smelling, toxic remains of undigested food that obstructs the channels in the body

apagni one of thefive ***bhutagnis***; it helps break down watery food

Apana Vata one of the five ***subdoshas*** of ***Vata***, governing all downward motion in the body, particularly in the lower abdomen

asanas neuromuscular integration exercises

asthi dhatu of the seven ***dhatus***, asthi is bone tissue

asthi agni one of the seven ***dhatu agnis***. The dhatu agnis transform one tissue into the other in the process of digestion.

Avalambaka Kapha one of the five ***subdoshas*** of ***Kapha***, centered in the chest, heart, and lower body; supports physical strength, the back, and stamina; regulates moisture in the lungs

Ayur-Veda "knowledge of life span"; a major category of Vedic Literature dealing with medicine and health

Bhrajaka Pitta one of the five ***subdoshas*** of ***Pitta***, associated with the skin, including appearance and absorptive activity

bhutagni general term for the five types of digestive fire (***agnis***) that correspond with each of the five elements of Nature (earth, water, fire, air, space) and help to digest foods according to the presence of those elements

Bodhaka Kapha one of the five ***subdoshas*** of ***Kapha***, located in the tongue and throat; regulates secretions in the mouth as well as the sense of taste

Charaka Samhita one of the 40 aspects of the Vedic Literature; the best known of the six aspects that deal explicitly with medicine and health

climacteric the biological change in all body tissue and systems that occurs in both sexes somewhere between the ages of 40 and 60

deha prakriti one's doshic constitution at any particular point in life (see ***dosha***, ***prakriti***)

dhatu any of the seven tissues that make up the body

dhatu agni digestive or metabolic fire associated with each of the seven bodily tissues

dosha any of the three fundamental operators underlying all aspects of the mind-body (see ***Vata***, ***Pitta***, and ***Kapha***)

dravyaguna "qualities of matter"; sophisticated science of preparing Ayurvedic herbal compounds

estrogen any of various natural steroid hormones (such as estradiol) that are formed from androgen precursors, that are secreted chiefly by the ovaries, placenta, adipose tissue, and testes, and that stimulate the development of female secondary sex characteristics and promote the growth and maintenance of the female reproductive system

Gandharva Veda music of the ancient Vedic civilization; the eternal rhythms and melodies of Nature

ghee clarified butter

hysterectomy surgical removal of the uterus

jala the element of water (see ***mahabhuta***)

janma prakriti the type of mind-body constitution one is born with

jatharagni the primary digestive fire functioning in the digestive juices in the large and small intestines and the stomach, which are responsible for converting food into the nutrient plasma that nourishes all the cells and tissues throughout the body; made up of the five ***bhutagnis***

Jyotish aspect of Vedic Literature concerned with Vedic astrology

Kapha one of the three mind-body operators (***doshas***); governs physical structure, including bones, muscle, and the lymphatic system, and fluid balance; primarily situated in the chest; primary qualities: heavy, oily, slow, cold, steady, solid, dull, soft, sweet, and smooth

kayachikitsa "therapy of fire"—the field of internal medicine used in Maharishi Rejuvenation therapy to sustain and balance the digestive fire (***agni***), including panchakarma and other procedures (such as ***abhyanga***) to purify and pacify the ***doshas***

Kledaka Kapha one of the five ***subdoshas*** of ***Kapha***, located in the stomach; responsible for the initial phases of digestion, especially moistening the food

mahabhuta any of the basic building blocks or elements of the materials world: earth (***prithivi***), water (***jala***), fire (***tejas***), air (***vayu***), and space (***akasha***).

Maharishi Ayur-Veda health care program Ayurvedic science of health and system of medicine revived in its completeness by Maharishi Mahesh Yogi

Maharishi Jyotish program science of prediction—Vedic astrology—revived in its completeness by Maharishi Mahesh Yogi

Maharishi Sthapatya Veda design aspect of Maharishi Vedic Science[SM] that includes the health effects of the orientation, design, proportion, and positioning of buildings; the most ancient and supreme system of country, town, village, and home planning in harmony with Natural Law

majja dhatu one of the seven ***dhatus***, majja includes bone marrow and the tissues of the nervous system

majja agni one of the seven ***dhatu agnis***. The dhatu agnis transform one tissue into the other in the process of digestion.

mala any of the several types of normal waste produced during formation of the ***dhatus***, including urine, feces, sweat, phlegm, bile, and various other excreta

mamsa dhatu of the seven ***dhatus***, mamsa is muscle tissue

mamsa agni one of the seven ***dhatu agnis***. The dhatu agnis transform one tissue into the other in the process of digestion.

meda dhatu of the seven ***dhatus***, meda is fat tissue

meda agni one of the seven ***dhatu agnis***. The dhatu agnis transform one tissue into the other in the process of digestion.

menopause the period of natural cessation of ***menstruation***

menstruation the cyclical ovarian process that begins in puberty in females

ojas the most refined and nourishing product of digestion; the finest material form of consciousness

osteoporosis a medical condition characterized by a loss of bone density; "brittle-bone" disease

Pachaka Pitta one of the five ***subdoshas*** of ***Pitta***, governing digestive secretions in the area of the small intestine, duodenum, and lower stomach

pandit an expert thoroughly trained to use Vedic technologies of sound and action to restore the functioning of Natural Law through, for example, the precise performances of ***yagyas***

perimenopause the years just before and just after a woman's last menstrual period

Pitta one of the three ***doshas***; governs heat, metabolism, and energy production; primarily situated in the area around the navel; primary qualities: hot, sharp, light, acidic, slightly oily, liquid and flowing

post-menopause the period of time starting a year after a woman's menstrual flow has stopped

pragya-aparadh "mistake of the intellect"

Prana Vata one of the five ***subdoshas*** of ***Vata***, governing movement of air, etc., in the head and chest, as well as mental clarity and sensory perception

pranayama neurorespiratory technique involving simple, rhythmic breathing exercises to balance, relax, and revitalize the mind-body

premenopause the years prior to the cessation of ***menstruation***

prithivi the element earth (see ***mahabhuta***)

prithivi agni one of the five ***bhutagnis***; it helps break down heavy , solid foods

progesterone a female steroid sex hormone that is secreted to prepare the uterus for pregnancy

raga musical patterns (melodies) structured according to the principles of ***Gandharva Veda*** music

rakta dhatu of the seven ***dhatus***, rakta equates with blood

rakta agni one of the seven ***dhatu agnis***. The dhatu agnis transform one tissue into the other in the process of digestion.

Ranjaka Pitta one of the ***subdoshas*** of ***Pitta***, governing blood chemistry and color from the liver and spleen

rasa essence or taste

rasa dhatu of the seven ***dhatus***, rasa is associated with chyle, or plasma, and is the first product of digestion

rasa agni one of the seven ***dhatu agnis***. The dhatu agnis transform one tissue into the other in the process of digestion.

rishi wise person, enlightened teacher

Sadhaka Pitta one of the five ***subdoshas*** of ***Pitta***, located in the heart and associated with desiring, fulfilling desires, memory, enthusiasm and energy

samadoshas a rare mind-body type characterized by a balance of all three ***doshas—Vata***, ***Pitta***, and ***Kapha***

Sama Veda one of the four ***Vedas*** (Ṛk, Sama, Yajur, and Atharva), whose frequencies express the "flowing wakefulness" quality of Natural Law

Samana Vata one of the five ***subdoshas*** of ***Vata***, located in the umbilical region; associated with appetite, production of digestive enzymes, and movement of food through the stomach and intestines

Shleshaka Kapha one of the five ***subdoshas*** of ***Kapha***, responsible for the lubrication of the joints

shukra the subtlest of the seven ***dhatus***; reproductive tissues

srota channels and microchannels within the body, such as veins, arteries and capillaries

Sthapatya Veda aspect of Vedic Literature concerned with architecture

Surya Namaskara "salute to the sun"—a special sequence of ***asanas***, or neuromuscular integration exercises

Tarpaka Kapha one of the five ***subdoshas*** of ***Kapha***, located in the head and cerebrospinal fluid; responsible for nourishing and lubricating the organs of the head and for nourishing the sensory and cognitive faculties, and motor organs

tejas the element of fire, also called agni (see ***mahabhuta***)

tejasagni one of the five ***bhutagnis***; it helps break down spicy or hot foods

Udana Vata one of the five ***subdoshas*** of ***Vata***, located in the throat, chest and navel

vastu the correct relationship between a building site and the environment

Vata the "king" of the three mind-body operators (***doshas***), because it leads ***Pitta*** and ***Kapha*** in responding to internal and external factors; governs motion of all kinds—mental, physical, emotional—from its primary seat in the colon; primary qualities: light, dry, cold, airy, moving, and consciousness

Vata Kala term used in the Vedic texts to refer to the later years of a woman's life, characterized by wisdom and tranquility

vayu the element of air (see ***mahabhuta***)

Veda "knowledge"—total knowledge and structure of Natural Law expressed in unmanifest frequencies of sound that precede and produce the physical manifestation of the universe

vikriti a state of imbalance in the doshas characterized by an excess of one or more ***doshas***

Vyana Vata one of the five ***subdoshas*** of ***Vata***; governs circulation of the blood, lymph, and sweat, as well as nerve impulses promoting, for example, extension and contraction of muscles

yagyas Vedic performances which aim to transform the influences on one's life so as to correct imbalances before they arise

INDEX

Page numbers with definitions are in italics.

About the Authors

Dr. Kumuda Reddy and **Dr. Janardhan Reddy** are a married team committed to bringing the time-tested knowledge of Maharishi Vedic Medicine to the modern world. Both are medical doctors with over 30 years of experience each in the practice of conventional western medicine. Trained in Maharishi Vedic Medicine, they have found that this natural, holistic system complements western care and has the potential to solve many of the health problems we face today.

Dr. Kumuda Reddy completed her residency and fellowship at Mt. Sinai Hospital, New York. For many years she was a faculty member at Albany Medical College. For the past ten years she has practiced Maharishi Vedic Medicine in upstate New York. She is in private practice in Bethesda, Maryland.

She previously coauthored three books on Maharishi Vedic Medicine: *Forever Healthy: Introduction to Maharishi Ayur-Veda Health Care, For a Blissful Baby: Healthy and Happy Pregnancy with Maharishi Vedic Medicine* and *Conquering Chronic Disease through Maharishi Vedic Medicine.* She also coauthored a book of stories from the Upanishads entitled *All Love Flows to the Self* and a series of children's stories called the *Timeless Wisdom Series,* based on traditional Indian stories that she first heard as a child.

Dr. Janardhan Reddy has extensive experience in various clinical fields, including urology, general surgery and neurosurgery. He completed his residency in urology and was in urological private practice for almost two decades.

Together, this husband-and-wife medical team write and give lectures on Maharishi Vedic Medicine. Their forthcoming books include *Living Life Free from Pain: Treating Joint Pain and Arthritis, Muscle Pain and Fibromyalgia with Maharishi Vedic Medicine* and a series of cookbooks titled *Not Everyone Needs the Same Kind of Food.*

The Reddys are active community members and devoted to their extended family. They have three children: Sundeep, Hima and Suma. They live and work in Rockville, Maryland.

Sandra Willbanks has her master's degree in professional writing from Maharishi University of Management in Fairfield, Iowa and has written plays, movies, and radio shows. A former newspaper correspondent, she specializes in writing about all aspects of health with an emphasis on Maharishi Vedic Medicine. She also writes a column for the *Iowa Source*, a monthly news magazine.

Questions and Answers: Addressing Common Concerns

Before the questions and answers I wish to convey to the readers that Maharishi Vedic Medicine is a traditional system of comprehensive medicine. Trying to treat one symptom at a time, like most modern practitioners do, is defeating the whole purpose. Just as I respect the tradition and I advocate it in my practice, so should the readers use this traditional system in its holistic and comprehensive form.

An experienced physician trained in Maharishi Vedic Medicine is necessary to put all the loose ends together and come up with solutions that can be easily followed and are compliant with Maharishi Vedic Medicine. Otherwise, Maharishi Vedic Medicine is so vast and deep in its knowledge that it only leads to confusion, and partial treatments can result. There are many things that one can do in small ways once the problems are addressed and resolved and the body is on the way to recovery. Ultimately the goal is to have self-sufficiency, and Maharishi Vedic Medicine allows self-sufficiency to develop in a spontaneous and effortless way, whereby one becomes intuitive to one's own body's needs. The overall benefit is a long, healthy and happy life.

Q. How difficult is this program to follow? As I read the book I see that there are many things that are of value and can be used, but it seems like a very big program that could be time-consuming.

A. There are over forty modalities in Maharishi Vedic Medicine, but we only choose a very few modalities to start with. For example, you can start with the diet and some herbs. It is the role of the experienced Ayurvedic physician to see what is most needed in each individual's case and what the patient can deal with.

Q. I like what I read and know about Maharishi Vedic Medicine, but I worry if I can be faithful to it. What do you advise?

A. *I think that there are three important factors: the desire to have this natural, holistic medicine; a good, experienced physician to help fulfill that desire; and some effort and faith on the patient's part.*

Q. I seem to have so many symptoms. Can they all be addressed?

A. *Maharishi Vedic Medicine, being holistic, recognizes that disease starts at the level of the source where there is the disconnection or mistake at the level of the body's inner intelligence. Then disease localizes in an organ or tissues and then spreads to other organs and systems. So when one is able to treat from that level of the source then it is possible to eliminate all the symptoms in one stroke.*

Q. Do some symptoms take longer to be treated than others?

A. *Yes. In the process of disease there are some imbalances that start earlier on and then reach other doshas, dhatus, srotas and malas. So in this sequential process there will be a delay of the onset of some of the symptoms. In the same process as the healing begins and the body's inner intelligence is enlivened, some symptoms disappear or go away much more quickly than the others.*

Q. How important is it that a person seeks Maharishi Vedic Medicine at the onset of disease?

A. *We understand that disease is also structured in layers. It becomes chronic and imbalances become deeper. When many organs and tissues become involved then the disease becomes more complicated. So that's why we recognize that it is important that we treat disease in early and moderate stages so that complete recovery is possible.*

Q. What happens if I cannot tolerate the foods or herbs that are recommended?

A. *The proper foods and herbs are recommended by taking into consideration the patient's condition. A physician trained in Maharishi Vedic Medicine would know how best to incorporate the program*

Q. Where are estrogens found naturally?

A. They are found in soy products, cashews, oats, corn, wheat, apples, almonds, lentils, pomegranates, lox, dairy products and a host of others. Estrogens are not hard to come by.

Q. Why is taking estrogens from an artificial source harmful?

A. When anything is taken from an outside artificial source it actually does not correlate and coordinate with the body's biological intelligence. The body uses foods and spices in a natural format and breaks them down, metabolizes and assimilates them. Then it releases nutrients in the body as needed. When you present anything from the outside in the form of pills, capsules or synthetic chemicals the body's intelligence becomes distorted and confused because it can't determine how much of the artificial substance the body needs, if any. It may flush out the substance altogether, or it may store it away, increasing the risk of disease later on.

Q. Do we really need hormones, such as Hormone Replacement Therapy, from an outside source for the rest of our lives?

A. No. The body's natural cycles are programmed in such a way that hormones are diminished at a certain age. This hormonal cycle is very delicate and intricate. Interfering with nature's process can result in long-term and serious consequences, some of which we know and some of which we are yet to discover.

Q. Do you recommend hormones at all?

A. If the patient has a very stormy onset of menopause where she's not able to handle the symptoms, then a short-term course of hormones, lasting for a few months or even a year or two depending on the need, is okay. This is crisis intervention and management, but it is not the long-term cure. Once you feel stronger then it's good to think in long-term use of Maharishi Vedic Medicine. Even during this process I would recommend that the Maharishi Ayurvedic process is started because it makes it easier.

Q. I'm going through perimenopause, and I seem to be having irregular and sometimes heavy periods. Why?

A. This is again due to hormonal imbalances that have been discussed in this book. The heavy periods are due to a Pitta dosha imbalance, etc. So when these are corrected you can handle perimenopause much more easily. In my experience I have found that most of these problems can be resolved with Maharishi Vedic Medicine very efficiently.

Q. I seem to experience fluid retention, much more than ever before. Is this my imagination?

A. This is an imbalance in Kapha and meda dhatu, which governs the body's balance of fluids. This can be addressed very well with the proper diet, exercise, and herbs.

Q. I wake up in the morning feeling stiff and achy. This is something new, I never had it before. Is this due to menopause?

A. Again, this is a Vata and Kapha imbalance. An imbalance in Rasa dhatu can give rise to body aches. A daily oil self-massage is part of balancing the doshas and srotas and will help keep the body subtle.

Q. I'm experiencing joint pain for the first time, mainly in my knees and hips. Why is that?

A. Most likely this can be the beginning of osteoarthritis and is a Vata imbalance. Vata regulates the nervous system and all movement in the body, and governs all sensory and motor activities. Osteoarthritis usually begins as a result of wear and tear on the joints during the latter part of life, and is characterized by a degenerative process in the joints. Even though all of the joints are vulnerable, the weight-bearing joints, such as the knee and hip, are most commonly involved. Arthritis involves whole systems of the body, and is not just located where the symptoms appear in the joints. The appearance of pain or joint stiffness is not the first stage of the disease but the fourth stage. In osteoarthritis aggravated Vata is associated with ama, a product of improper digestion. Consequently, the treatment includes alleviation of Vata, plus correction of other imbalances and correction of ama formation. With Maharishi Vedic Medicine we can prevent further progression.

Q. I seem to experience enormous fatigue and tiredness. I have never experienced anything like this before. I keep taking all kinds of vitamins and minerals. I don't have any energy to do an exercise program. Is the problem iron deficiency?

A. This is due to a Vata imbalance. Also, if you are obese or overweight it might be a Kapha imbalance. The srotas might be blocked. In my practice this can be fairly easily corrected.

Q. I feel very emotional and teary, and I cry over little things. My heart seems to be very sensitive. Why am I so emotional?

A. This can be due to an imbalance in the Sadhaka Pitta subdosha (emotional heart) and also in the Vata dosha. In my experience, using herbs and proper diet restores balance. Also the practice of the Transcendental Meditation technique and Maharishi Vedic Vibration Technology helps balance the emotions.

Q. I seem to go through a depression. When I get up in the morning I feel fine but when I go through the day I get depressed. It seems to come and go, and it disrupts my everyday existence. Am I really depressed?

A. This seems like more of a Kapha, Vata and Tamasic (inertia and dullness) imbalance. Menopause is the time of life governed by Vata. Because Vata is highly mobile and unstable, it is the most prone of the three doshas to be aggravated. When Vata is out of balance or there is too much Vata in a woman's physiology, Vata can manifest as unfounded fear, worry, insomnia and loneliness, which may lead to depressing thoughts. A key to eliminating any physiological or psychological discomfort associated with the transition into menopause is to balance the functioning of Vata dosha. Maharishi Vedic Medicine has many ways of avoiding these out-of-balance Vata symptoms through healthy eating habits (for your body type), specific herbs and proper daily routine.

Q. I have a long-standing depression that doesn't seem to lift. I have taken an anti-depression medication but it doesn't relieve my problem. I have no interest in life around me and I just drag through the day. Can depression be helped without drugs?

A. This seems more like a Kapha and Tamas imbalance, which leads to inertia and dullness in thinking. It's important to remember that the dhatus and srotas can be involved. It's okay to be on conventional medicine if it is helping, and we can add Maharishi Vedic Medicine as a compleiment to it. Or, for many people the holistic approach of Maharishi Vedic Medicine seems to be enough.

Q. I'm having feelings of enormous anger. Every little thing bothers me and I have developed a short fuse. Why do little things anger me so much?

A. This is clearly an imbalance in Pitta dosha. Conventional medicine can do very little to help with this. But Maharishi Vedic Medicine, by balancing the mind, body and emotions, can bring calmness to the mind and peace to the heart. Again several techniques like eating the proper food, herbs and spices, and practicing meditation and the Maharishi Vibrational Technology technique, are all helpful.

Q. I feel very overwhelmed in life. I can't seem to organize myself or handle the jobs that I'm confronted with. I feel panicky, anxious, and confused. Is this what menopause is like?

A. This is again a Vata imbalance, and many of the techniques used to balance Vata end up bringing harmony and integration to the nervous system. This feeling of being overwhelmed may have happened periodically during your life, and then it seems to get aggravated again during menopause because Vata takes over at this time of life.

Q. I have a hard time remembering names, faces and events. Sometimes I feel that I am losing my mind. I'm told that I have to take HRT for this. Am I now coming down with Alzheimer's?

A. Some loss of memory happens gradually with the aging process, but it should not be all of a sudden and rapidly progressing. Maharishi Vedic Medicine has many herbs and techniques, such as Transcendental Meditation, panchakarma and Maharishi Vedic Vibration Technology, that are strengthening, rejuvenating and revitalizing to the nervous system, establishing integrity and harmony. There are also modalities that clear the communication of the srotas and there are herbs for the brain that improve oxygenation and circulation.

Q. My hot flashes do not respond to anything that I take. What should I do?

A. Imbalances happen over a long period of time. In Maharishi Vedic Medicine it says imbalances start to accumulate at the time of conception. If they are not treated and balanced periodically, they become chronic and aggravated. If the imbalances are not treated over time then the treatment may take a longer time, perhaps a few months.

Q. Do hot flashes and other menopausal symptoms last forever?

A. In general they seem to last for a few months or a few years. That's why HRT for the rest of your life is not an appropriate treatment. With Maharishi Vedic Medicine this course of discomfort and agony can be cut short and eliminated completely. In Maharishi Vedic Medicine too much heat in the body is known to be produced by an imbalance of Pitta dosha. Maharishi Vedic Medicine herbal supplements along with a balanced diet and mild purification will help relieve symptoms. A physician trained in Maharishi Ayur-Veda may also recommend special foods or drinks that are correct for your constitution and will help with hot flashes.

Q. I'm experiencing heat in the body, but it's not like a hot flash. What is it?

A. This heat is a variation of a hot flash, caused by an imbalance in the Bhrajaka Pitta dosha. Again, the imbalances are usually accumulated over a period of many years but can be treated with Maharishi Vedic Medicine.

Q. I seem to experience tension headaches. I feel tense all day and experience tension headaches on an everyday basis. I use to get an occasional headache before I went into menopause, but now they seem to be regular. What causes this?

A. Tension headaches are usually a Vata imbalance. Both the Prana Vata and Vyana Vata are disturbed. The lack of proper rest and imbalances in the nervous system can cause these. They usually respond very well with the regular Maharishi Vedic Medicine treatments.

Q. I used to get an occasional migraine headache when I was younger. But now I seem to be getting them on a weekly basis, and they have disrupted my life. I feel exhausted with pain and nausea. Can Maharishi Vedic Medicine help?

A. Migraine headaches are a disturbance in the Pitta and Vata doshas. I have found that many patients do not respond to conventional medicine, or they have to take a lot of conventional medicine, which makes them very ill with side effects. Patients with this problem respond well to Maharishi Vedic Medicine.

Q. There is a history of heart disease in my family. My mother died of a heart attack and my father died of a stroke. My doctor says I should take HRT to prevent heart disease. Will taking HRT prevent my having a heart attack?

A. It's important to recognize that manifestations of heart disease like high blood pressure, high cholesterol, blocking of the arteries, etc. starts long before menopause. In Maharishi Vedic Medicine we recognize that these signs can start accumulating as early as the second and third decades of life. It sounds inappropriate when someone says that HRT will prevent all heart disease. It may give some protection, but it's not foolproof.

Q. What are the treatments you have in Maharishi Vedic Medicine that prevent heart disease?

A. Imbalances can be in all the three doshas. People with a Vata imbalance are prone to hypertension. People with a Pitta imbalance are prone to type B heart disease—angina and heart attacks—because of their lifestyles and emotional tendencies towards anger and irritability. Kapha people tend to have heart disease because of weight gain, increased cholesterol, abnormal lipids and clogging of the arteries. Maharishi Vedic Medicine prevents and treats heart disease accordingly by balancing the doshas, building and rejuvenating the dhatus, cleaning the srotas, and using rasayanas, which strengthen the cardiovascular system as a whole. In this context, the food, exercise and meditation are all necessary and vital components, in addition to regular panchakarma treatments.

Q. Are there any rasayanas for the heart that can be used on a regular basis for the rest of my life?

A. Yes, there are extremely good rasayanas for the heart that can be recommended and used on a regular basis. They are good for both prevention and correction of the imbalances as and when they arise.

Q. I've been told to take HRT to prevent osteoporosis. Is this good to take?

A. Again in Maharishi Vedic Medicine we realize that osteoporosis can start as early as the mid-twenties and become progressive, especially if one does not know how to take care of oneself in preventing or halting this disease. So HRT started at the time of menopause or after menopause provides very little help compared to the many side effects it produces. In Maharishi Vedic Medicine we recognize that each one is susceptible to this in a unique and individual way. The thin-boned and thin-framed Vata mind/body types are more prone to osteoporosis than the medium-build Pittas and the large-boned Kaphas. Maharishi Vedic Medicine gives a wide variety of treatments for both prevention and treatment without any side effects.

Q. What are the diets that contain calcium?

A. Dark green leafy vegetables such as as collard greens, spinach, mustard greens, bok choy greens, and many varieties of kale are sources of calcium. Eat them every day. Also nuts (almonds, sunflower seeds, Brazil nuts, sesame seeds), legumes (tofu, garbanzo beans, pinto beans, etc.), dairy products (lassi, yogurt, milk) all contain calcium. Maharishi Vedic Medicine recommends special natural supplements, herbs and minerals that can be taken to help with calcium absorption. There are special preparations that actually increase bone density and bone regeneration. In my practice these have been equally as effective as Fosamax, which can have many unwanted side- effects. Exercise also plays an important role in maintaining bone density. (See the chapter on exercise).

Q. Dr. Reddy, do you say that one cannot use these pharmaceutical products for increasing bone density at all?

A. If there is an acute situation where one needs to intervene rapidly and also in spinal compression fractures, yes these can be used for a shorter period of time. But I'm not sure if they offer any advantage, if used over a longer period of time, over the naturally available Maharishi Vedic Medicine preparations.

Q. Are there any more tips you can give on performing yoga asanas?

A. Performing yoga asanas should be easy and effortless. Therefore, never strain or force yourself into any pose. Practicing yoga asanas is not a competitive sport, so go at your own unhurried pace. Because it is an exercise, don't eat right before practicing your yoga asana routine. And make sure you rest before continuing your day.

Q. What is the best time to practice yoga asanas?

A. It is ideal to start your day with yoga asanas followed by the practice of the Transcendental Meditation technique and to repeat the routine after your workday but before your evening starts. However, performing a few yoga stretches during the day will help keep you flexible and limber.

Q. Are there more yoga stretches that I can do?

A. There are hundreds of yoga asanas and many different teachers who teach them. However, many of these teachers, especially in the west, do not have a complete understanding of how the postures should be performed. Therefore, I recommend that you find a teacher who is trained in Maharishi Yoga Asanas, because this person can give you a correct routine. (For a teacher in your area see the appendix.)

Q. I have been experiencing acne for the first time since being a teenager. Is this normal at menopause?

A. This is due to the Pitta dosha and subdoshas being out of balance. Ranjaka Pitta is in charge of balanced liver function, pure blood cells, and cell nutrition, and Bhrajaka Pitta regulates skin temperature and the healthy glow of the skin. Acne can also appear because the channels of circulation are blocked. Maharishi

Vedic Medicine has the comprehensive program of diet, special herbs, skin preparations and other modalities to eliminate this problem very quickly.

Q. I'm experiencing age spots. What causes them?

A. It's usually imbalances in Vata and Pitta and also on the level of the srotas. As you age the skin becomes dryer and thinner, which is Vata- related, and more sensitive to the sun, which is due to Bhrajaka Pitta becoming more active. Improper diet can show up on the back of the hands as age spots or "liver spots" caused by the excess of Vata that arrives with aging. Maharishi Vedic Medicine has special skin treatments, including herbalized oils and lotions, that help with aging skin, along with special dietary recommendations.

Q. I have developed a very dry skin with flaky patches. How do I get rid of this condition?

A. Dry skin is due to an imbalance in Vyana Vata (which is the subdosha of Vata that governs circulation and sensitivity, affecting proper nourishment) and in Rasa dhatu. An imbalanced Bhrajaka Pitta also has a drying effect. Together they affect Shleshaka Kapha, which governs moisture balance and lubrication. Dry patches could be the beginning of eczema, but these problems can be resolved very quickly with Maharishi Vedic Medicine oil massage and other recommendations that are especially beneficial to the skin.

Q. I'm having cracking in my nails. They seem to break off easily and they are very brittle. And some of my toes seem to be discolored. What can I do?

A. Brittle nails are caused by Rasa dhatu and Ashti dhatu imbalances that need to be corrected. Discoloration in the nail beds is usually due to fungus, which has to be treated properly.

Q. I'm experiencing hair loss with a dry and sometimes flaky scalp. What natural method can I use to change this?

A. Some hair loss is normal with the aging process. But rapid hair loss should be a concern. This condition is due to imbalances in Vata and Ashti dhatu, which when imbalanced causes falling hair, nails and teeth, and loose joints. Stress, poor diet, hormone imbalance, excessive sun and harsh chemicals in shampoos, can all have a damaging effect on hair. In my practice, with the proper diagnosis and treatment, this problem has been helped with many patients.

Q. I seem to have frequency of urination more so during the night. I feel like I'm waking up every hour. Is this part of menopause?

A. This is a fairly common problem around and during menopause due to an Apana Vata imbalance. The malas or body waste (urine) can be affected by imbalances in the srotas, doshas and dhatus. HRT has also been recommended for this problem but in my practice I have treated it very quickly and successfully with Maharishi Vedic Medicine.

Q. I seem to have an urgency to urinate and if I don't empty my bladder immediately there seems to be leakage. Is this normal?

A. This is due to an imbalance in Apana Vata, which is located in the bladder as well as other places. If this is a recent problem, it is fairly easily corrected with Maharishi Vedic Medicine. If it's a long-standing problem, there may be some other pathology that needs medical attention.

Q. I have been experiencing frequent urinary tract infections. Every time I'm put on antibiotics I feel very rundown and I get candida infections in my genital area. I'm told to take HRT to prevent this. What does Maharishi Vedic Medicine recommend?

A. Frequent urinary tract infections are again due to an imbalance in Apana Vata and Pitta, and also to lowered immunity. This cycle can be ended very easily with Maharishi Vedic Medicine, without the agony of going through repeated courses of antibiotics and being exposed to their side effects.

Q. I feel a dull discomfort in my bladder area and am experiencing urinary hesitancy. It takes a long time to empty my bladder. Do I have to live with this?

A. This is an imbalance in the Apana Vata. It's good to rule out bladder cysts, stones, or tumors. I have had, in general, good response with these kinds of problems if there is no existing surgical pathology.

Q. I seem to have decreased libido. Is this normal at menopause?

A. This is usually a Vata and Pitta imbalance. The Shukra Dhatu is also involved. Most patients experience good vitality and restoration of their normal sexual function with Maharishi Vedic Medicine.

Q. When menopause started I experienced extreme fatigue. No matter what I take I don't seem to feel better. What can be done?

A. This is an imbalance in the Vata and Kapha doshas; in addition, the dhatus and rasas need to be rejuvenated and the srotas need to be cleared. In my practice I have found that, with a little effort on the patient's part, they come out of that unending cycle of fatigue.

Q. I'm not able to sleep because of hot flashes and urinary frequency. Do I just have to wait this out?

A. Sleep problems are frequent around menopause. Women with a predominance of Vata dosha have problems going to sleep, while Pitta mind/body types have problems with excess heat in the body, which results in hot flashes. Apana Vata needs to be addressed in regards to urinary frequency. These can all be balanced with Maharishi Vedic Medicine; then good sleep becomes possible.

Q. Do I have to take a lot of multi vitamins and minerals?

A. If you are having an acute deficiency of any vitamins, then vitamins taken in pill form can help for a short period of time. In the long run Maharishi Vedic Medicine works better with natural food substitutes and spices, which bring integrity and harmony to the body's inner intelligence so that it utilizes and assimilates the nutrients better. Anything in pill form is not well absorbed or uti-

lized and becomes a free radical, or ama, which becomes a source for future disease.

Q. Should I use co enzyme Q 10 or other supplements?

A. Maharishi Vedic Medicine works best when its own inner intelligence is enlivened and brought into harmony so that the body itself produces all the enzymes, secretions and hormonal and biochemical substances as is needed. Giving outside enzymes is part of a reductionistic approach whereby the body's natural enzymes and pathways are suppressed and can become totally dysfunctional and even nonfunctional. Taking any of these outside materials is like a shotgun approach and is only good for a short period of time. They are all right for a crisis situation but do not offer any long-term solutions to the existing problem, which is simply masked and ignored. We have the appropriate natural supplements in Maharishi Vedic Medicine.

Q. I feel a lot of anxiety, worry and loneliness. Is this due to menopause?

A. It's a Vata imbalance. To transcend this and gain inner strength and self-sufficiency is the goal of Maharishi Vedic Medicine.

Q. I understand that the menstrual cycle is a cleansing cycle. How is the body rejuvenated once this cycle stops?

A. With diet and herbs and other Maharishi Vedic Medicine technologies such as massage, the body can be rejuvenated on a regular basis. Massage forms a part of the Ayurvedic purification and rejuvenation program called panchakarma, and these special massage routines are performed by qualified therapists under the supervision of a physician trained in Maharishi Vedic Medicine. Panchakarma is profoundly effective in bringing greater balance and rejuvenation in a very short span of time.

Q. Exactly how does panchakarma help in this situation?

A. The menstrual cycle is a natural way for a woman's body to cleanse itself every month. Panchakarma cleanses and enlivens the body through the senses, nervous system and circulation. It pacifies Vata by lubricating the physiology, purifying the channels, and maintaining the flow of the intellect in all areas of the physiology. When the menstrual cycle stops a woman especially needs some way to purify her body. Daily oil self-massage helps the body cleanse on a daily basis. However, toxins can accumulate over time. Panchakarma is a way to thoroughly remove toxins from the deeper levels of the body, which helps slow down the aging process. A physician trained in Maharishi Vedic Medicine will make recommendations as to the types of cleansing treatments given depending on the person's needs.

Q. How frequently should one take panchakarma?

A. It is recommended that one should take panchakarma twice a year at the seasonal change, or as needed. There are different types and lengths of programs that use various methods for cleansing and rejuvenation.